C. M. Witt, K. Linde

Clinical Research in Complementary and Integrative Medicine

A Practical Training Book

Claudia M. Witt, Klaus Linde

Clinical Research in Complementary and Integrative Medicine

A Practical Training Book

1. Edition

In collaboration with Adrian White, Plymouth, UK

Preface by George Lewith and Brian Berman

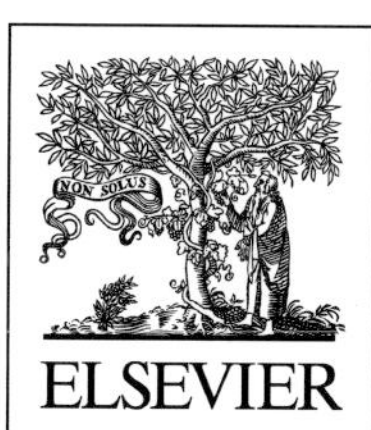

All business correspondence should be made with:
Elsevier GmbH, Urban & Fischer Verlag, Lektorat Integrative und Komplementäre Medizin, Hackerbrücke 6, 80335 Munich, Germany

Notice for the reader:
While reasonable efforts have been made to ensure that the guidance given in this book is factually correct, we cannot guarantee the completeness and that it can be applied to your study. This book aims to provide a basic introduction and further readings of more specialized literature and expert advice will be necessary to carry out your research. The case studies used in this book are fictitious.

Bibliographic information published by the Deutsche Nationalbibliothek
The Deutsche Nationalbibliothek lists this publication in the Deutsche Nationalbibliografie; detailed bibliographic data are available in the Internet at http://www.d-nb.de.

11 12 13 14 15 5 4 3 2 1

Acquisition Editor: Martina Braun, Munich
Development Editor: Bettina Lunk, Munich
Formal Editor: Ute Villwock, Heidelberg
Production Manager: Ulrike Schmidt, Munich
Composed by: abavo GmbH, Buchloe/Germany; TnQ, Chennai/India
Printed and bound by: L.E.G.O. S.p.A., Lavis/Italy
Illustrations: Stefan Dangl, Munich
Comics: Erik Liebermann, Steingaden
Cover Design: SpieszDesign, Neu-Ulm

ISBN: 978-0-7020-3476-3

Current information by **www.elsevier.de** and **www.elsevier.com**

Preface

The last 30 years have seen a well documented increase in the provision of Complementary and Alternative Medicine (CAM) throughout the industrialized Western countries. Within the EU, we estimate that there are now approximately 100 million CAM users and accurate data from the United States, the United Kingdom and Europe suggest that at least 15 % of the population is using CAM each year with over 50 % being lifetime users. This places a clear onus on medical researchers, politicians and indeed the public finances to develop thoughtful, cogent research strategies that will allow us to understand the reasons behind the popularity of CAM as well as its safety and effectiveness. Without this evidence it would be inappropriate to integrate new techniques in current healthcare provision.

We need to understand why it has become so popular. Who is providing it and how and why it is perceived to be beneficial by intelligent, educated and well-informed individuals? We need better evidence and less „conviction politics" in order for us to make rational decisions about the public and private provision of CAM. In order to do this we need a thoughtful and educated group of researchers who can develop and inform our understanding of these diverse therapies. This will allow us to understand exactly what it is about CAM that some people perceive as helpful, while at the same time learning how we may integrate the best medical provision from both conventional and complementary medicine into a patient-centered and integrated package.

Witt and Linde established their summer research training course[1] in 2007 to develop and improve scientific knowledge within this field and to foster more research within CAM. This allows us to move away from the position of being poorly informed and self-opinionated when considering CAM towards an improved understanding of the strengths and weaknesses within this area of medicine. Their book provides an excellent, thought-provoking and meticulous set of guidelines for constructing a variety of different study interventions to allow us to evaluate CAM. Above all else Witt and Linde's approach is grounded in practical experience and simple practical common sense thus making the information easy to access and use. CAM is widely available and therefore represents a potential public health hazard as well as a significant and often hidden element of our health service provision.

It has been suggested that CAM provision in the United States is responsible for far greater out of pocket expenditure than conventional medicine[2]. As a consequence, medical researchers and research funders have a duty of care to their populations to enable the creation of a thoughtful and appropriate evaluative culture within this field. Witt and Linde have made a very clear, concise and substantial contribution to research development in this area as a consequence of their summer school and we hope that this new publication, which summarizes their approach, will be widely read and valued by all those interested in this particular area of medicine.

September 2010
George Lewith
Brian Berman

[1] Witt CM, Linde K. The need of CAM research training. Forsch Komplementärmed Klass Naturheilkd 2008; 15: 69-70.

[2] Eisenberg DM, Davis RB, and Ettner SL. Trends in alternative medicine use in the United States. JAMA 1998; 280: 246–52.

We would like to thank

Robert Bosch Stiftung
Iris Bartsch
Daniela Hacke
Christine Holmberg
Ania Kania
Christl Kiener
Rainer Lüdtke
Sossie Kassab
Stefanie Roll
Andrew Vickers
Adrian White

Glossary

Adjusted analysis
Usually refers to attempts to control (adjust) for baseline imbalances in important patient characteristics.
Sometimes used to refer to adjustments of p-value to take account of multiple testing. [1]

Adverse event (AE)
Any adverse change in health or side effect that occurs in a person who participates in a study. AEs are classified as serious (➢ SAE) or minor; expected or unexpected; and study-related, possibly study-related, or not study-related.

Allocation concealment
A technique used to prevent selection bias by concealing the allocation sequence from those assigning participants to intervention groups, until the moment of assignment. Allocation concealment prevents researchers from (unconsciously or otherwise) influencing which participants are assigned to a given intervention group. [1]

Attrition
See loss to follow-up

Bias
Systematic distortion of the estimated intervention effect away from the „truth", caused by inadequacies in the design, conduct or analysis of a trial. [1]

Blinding
The practice of keeping the trial participants, care providers, those collecting data, and sometimes even those analyzing data unaware of which intervention is being administered to which participant. Blinding is intended to prevent bias on the part of study personnel. The most common application is „double-blinding", in which participants, caregivers and those assessing outcome are blinded to intervention assignment. The term „masking" may be used instead of blinding. [1]

Block randomization
An approach to generating an allocation sequence in which the number of assignments to intervention groups satisfies a specified allocation ratio (such as 1 : 1 or 2 : 1) after every „block" of specified size.
For example, a block of size 12 would contain 6 A and 6 B with a ratio of 1 : 1 or 8 A and 4 B with a ratio of 2 : 1. Generating the allocation sequence involves randomly selecting from all the permutations of assignments that meet the specified ratio. [1]

Case Report Form (CRF)
All data on each patient participating in a clinical trial are held and/or documented in the CRF. This can be on paper or in an electronic file.

Categorical variable
A categorical variable is one that has two or more categories.

Clinical research
Clinical research is a branch of medical science that determines the safety and effectiveness of medications, devices, diagnostic products and treatment regimens intended for human use. These may be used for prevention, treatment, diagnosis or for relieving symptoms of a disease. [2]

Clinical trial
An experiment to compare the effects of two or more healthcare interventions.
Clinical trial is an umbrella term for a variety of designs of healthcare trials, including uncontrolled trials, controlled trials, and randomised controlled trials. [1]

Cluster randomization
In a trial using cluster randomization it is not the individual patient who is randomized to group A or B but a group or cluster of patients. For example, 25 practices (and all their patients meeting the inclusion criteria) are randomized to group A and 25 practices to group B.

Co-intervention
Application of additional diagnostic and/or therapeutic procedures to participants in the trial.

Continuous variable
A continuous variable is one for which, within the limits of the variable's range, any value is possible.

Comparative effectiveness research
The generation and synthesis of evidence that compares the benefits and harms of alternative methods to prevent, diagnose, treat, and monitor a clinical condition or to improve the delivery of care. The purpose of CER is to assist consumers, clinicians, purchasers, and policy makers to make informed decisions that will improve health care at both the individual and population levels. [5]

Confounding
A situation in which the intervention effect is biased because of some difference between the comparison groups apart from the planned interventions, such as baseline characteristics, prognostic factors, or concomitant interventions. For a factor to be a confounder, it must differ between the comparison groups and predict the outcome of interest. [1]

CONSORT
The CONSORT Statement is intended to improve the reporting of a randomized controlled trial, enabling readers to understand a trial's design, conduct, analysis and interpretation, and to assess the validity of its results. [10]

Cross-sectional study
Cross-sectional studies (also known as Cross-sectional analysis) form a class of research methods that involve observation of a whole population, or a representative subset, at a defined time. [2]

Declaration of Helsinki
A statement of ethical principles for medical research involving human subjects, including research on identifiable human material and data developed by the The World Medical Association. [11]

Diagnostic reliability study
Diagnostic reliability studies investigate whether several investigators independently reach the same conclusion when applying a diagnostic test (inter-rater reliability), or whether the same investigator comes to the same conclusion at different times (intra-rater reliability).
Diagnostic validity study
Studies of diagnostic validity (or diagnostic accuracy) investigate whether a diagnostic procedure is helpful to rule in or rule out a diagnosis. They typically compare the diagnostic procedure of interest with the best method of establishing a diagnosis (comparison with gold standard).
Double-dummy technique
A technique to achieve blinding in clinical studies where two active treatments are being compared, the modes of administration of which are very different or cannot be matched. E.g. in a trial one group of patients could receive true acupuncture and placebo drug while the other group receives sham acupuncture and the true drug treatment.
Effect size
A measure of the difference in outcome between intervention groups. Commonly expressed as a risk ratio (relative risk), odds ratio or risk difference for binary outcomes and as difference in means for continuous outcomes. Often referred to as the „effect size". [1]
Effectiveness
Effectiveness is a measure of the extent to which a specific intervention when deployed in the field in routine circumstances does what it is intended to do for a specific population. [6]
Efficacy
Efficacy refers to the extent to which a specific intervention is beneficial under ideal conditions. [6]
Epidemiology
Epidemiology is the study of patterns of health and illness and associated factors at the population level. [2]
Evidence-based medicine
Evidence based medicine is the conscientious, explicit, and judicious use of current best evidence in making decisions about the care of individual patients. The practice of evidence based medicine means integrating individual clinical expertise with the best available external clinical evidence from systematic research. [3]
Explanatory trials
Trials designed to test causal research hypotheses – for example, that an intervention causes a particular biological change – are called explanatory. [7]
External validity
The extent to which the results of a trial provide a correct basis for generalizations to other circumstances. Also called „generalizability" or „applicability". [1]
Good Clinical Practice (GCP) Guideline
The GCP document describes the responsibilities and expectations of all participants in the conduct of clinical trials, including investigators, monitors, sponsors and IRBs. [9]
Health services research
Health services research is the multidisciplinary field of scientific investigation that studies how social factors, financing systems, organizational structures and processes, health technologies, and personal behaviours affect access to health care, the quality and cost of health care, and quantity and quality of life. Studies in health services research examine outcomes at the individual, family, organizational, institutional, community, and population level. HSR studies examine how people get access to health care, how much care costs, and what happens to patients as a result of this care. [4]
The incremental cost-effectiveness ratio (ICER)
The ICER represents the additional cost of one unit of outcome gained by a healthcare intervention or strategy, when compared to the next best alternative, mutually exclusive intervention or strategy. The ICER is calculated by dividing the net cost of the intervention by the total number of incremental health outcomes prevented by the intervention.
Impure placebo
A pharmacological active substance that has no specific effect on the disease under study
Intention to treat analysis
A strategy for analyzing data in which all participants are included in the group to which they were assigned, whether or not they completed the intervention given to the group. Intention-to-treat analysis prevents bias caused by the loss of participants, which may disrupt the baseline equivalence established by random assignment and which may reflect non-adherence to the protocol. [1]
Internal validity
The extent to which the design and conduct of the trial eliminate the possibility of bias. [1]
IRB/Ethics committee
Institutional Review Boards (IRB) or ethics committees are formally designated to approve, monitor, and review research in humans and animals to protect their rights and welfare.
Loss to follow-up
The circumstance that occurs when researchers lose contact with some participants and thus cannot complete planned data collection efforts. A common cause of missing data, especially in long-term studies. [1]
Matching
Matching is a procedure which aims to reduce differences between groups by forming pairs or sub-groups of patients who are identical or as similar as possible for relevant factors with regards to prognosis (e.g., age, gender, disease severity).
Meta-analysis
A (→) systematic review is called a meta-analysis if it includes an integrative statistical analysis (pooling) of the results of the included studies
Minimization
An assignment strategy, similar in intention to stratification, that ensures excellent balance between intervention

groups for specified prognostic factors. The next participant is assigned to whichever group would minimize the imbalance between groups on specified prognostic factors. Minimization is an acceptable alternative to random assignment. [1]

N-of-1 trial

Experiment in a single patient in which two or more different treatment options (e.g. true treatment and placebo) are repeatedly applied in a randomized order

Patient centred outcomes

Outcomes important to patients have been called 'patient-centered' outcomes.

Power

The probability that a trial will detect, as statistically significant, an intervention effect of a specified size. The pre-specified trial size is often chosen to give the trial the desired power. [1]

Pragmatic trials

Trials designed to help choose between different options for care are called pragmatic. [7]

Publication bias

Selective non-publication or delayed publication of undesired (often negative) findings

Pure placebo

A pharmacologically inactive substance

Quality adjusted life year (QALY)

This is a unit commonly used to measure health gain where the duration of the survival is adjusted by the patients' quality of life by multiplying the duration of survival with a utility weight that represents the quality of life of the health state experienced during that time.

Randomization

In a randomized trial, the process of assigning participants to groups such that each participant has a known and usually an equal chance of being assigned to a given group. Intended to ensure that the group assignment cannot be predicted. [1]

Randomized controlled trial

An experiment in which two or more interventions, possibly including a control intervention or no intervention, are compared by being randomly allocated to participants. In most trials one intervention is assigned to each individual but sometimes assignment is to defined groups of individuals (for example, in a household) or interventions are assigned within individuals (for example, in different orders or to different parts of the body). [1]

Reliability

Is the consistency of the results when a number of measurements are taken with the same measurement instrument.

Restricted randomization

Any procedure used with random assignment to achieve balance between study groups in size or baseline characteristics. Blocking is used to ensure that comparison groups will be of approximately the same size. With stratification, randomization with restriction is carried out separately within each of two or more subsets of participants (for example, defining disease severity or study centers) to ensure that the patient characteristics are closely balanced within each intervention group. [1]

Sample size

The number of participants in the trial. The intended sample size is the number of participants planned to be included in the trial, usually determined using a statistical power calculation. The sample size should be adequate to provide a high probability of detecting as significant an effect size of a given magnitude if such an effect actually exists. The achieved sample size is the number of participants enrolled, treated or analyzed in the study. [1]

Serious adverse Events (SAE)

Adverse events (➤ AE) categorized as 'serious' are called SAE. These are death, illness requiring hospitalization, events deemed life-threatening, or involving cancer or fetal exposure.

Sham procedure

A procedure mimicking a true intervention that has no specific effect on the disease under study

Stratification (syn. stratified randomization)

Random assignment within groups defined by participant characteristics, such as age or disease severity, intended to ensure good balance of these factors across intervention groups (see also ➤ Restricted randomization).

Systematic review

A review is called systematic if it uses predefined and explicit methods for identifying, selecting and assessing the information (typically research studies) that is considered relevant for answering a particular question posed.

Translational research

Translational research is a way of thinking about and conducting scientific research to make the results of research applicable to the population under study and is practised in the natural and biological, behavioural, and social sciences. [2] The idea is to transfer results from 'bench' to 'bedside.'

Validity

Refers to the extent to which a measurement, e.g. questionnaire, is well-founded and corresponds accurately to the real world.

Waiting list (or wait list) group control

A control group that is assigned to a waiting list to receive an intervention after the active treatment group does. A wait list control group serves the purpose of providing an untreated comparison for the active treatment group, while at the same time allowing the wait-listed participants an opportunity to obtain the intervention at a later date.

Whole Medical Systems

These are complete systems of theory and practice that have evolved over time in different cultures and apart from conventional or Western medicine. Examples systems include Ayurvedic medicine and traditional Chinese medicine and homeopathy. [8]

REFERENCES

[1] www.consort-statement.org/resources/glossary
[2] www.wikipedia.org/wiki/
[3] Sackett DL, Rosenberg WMC, Muir Gray JA, Haynes RB, Scott Richardson W. Evidence based medicine: what it is and what it isn't. BMJ 1996;312:71
[4] www.academyhealth.org/
[5] www.nap.edu/openbook.php?record_id=12648&page=29
[6] Last J, Spasoff, RA, Harris S: A Dictionary of Epidemiology. Oxford, Oxford University Press, 2001.
[7] Schwartz D, Lellouch J: Explanatory and pragmatic attitudes in therapeutical trials. J Chronic Dis 1967;20:637–648.
[8] www.nccam.nih.gov/health/whatiscam/
[9] www.ich.org/products/guidelines/efficacy/article/efficacy-guidelines.html
[10] www.consort-statement.org/
[11] www.wma.net/en/30publications/10policies/b3/index.html

Contents

CHAPTER

1 Introduction

1.1 What do we mean by complementary medicine in this book?

A variety of terms are used in public discussion about the heterogeneous collection of therapies whose evaluation methods will be discussed in this book. The most authoritative definitions come from the website (www.nccam.nih.gov/health/whatiscam; accessed January 2010) of the single most important research funding agency for research in the area, the US National Center of Complementary and Alternative Medicine (NCCAM):

- **Complementary and alternative medicine (CAM)** "is a group of diverse medical and health care systems, practices, and products that are not generally considered to be part of conventional medicine. While scientific evidence exists regarding some CAM therapies, for most there are key questions that are yet to be answered through well-designed scientific studies – questions such as whether these therapies are safe and whether they work for the purposes for which they are used."
- "**Complementary medicine** is used together with conventional medicine. An example of a complementary therapy is using aromatherapy to help lessen a patient's discomfort following surgery."
- "**Alternative medicine** is used in place of conventional medicine. An example of an alternative therapy is using a special diet to treat cancer instead of undergoing surgery, radiation, or chemotherapy that has been recommended by a conventional doctor."
- "**Integrative medicine** combines treatments from conventional medicine and CAM for which there is evidence of safety and effectiveness. It is also called integrated medicine."

It appears that patients are less interested in the details of terminology since the most commonly used term in the population is still alternative medicine. However, when asked about health care delivery, most patients prefer an approach with treatment options from both conventional and complementary medicine (Dobos 2009).

The perspective of providers is influenced by their own professional background. Practitioners are usually specialized in one particular complementary treatment (e.g. Chinese medicine, homeopathy), in contrast to physicians (i.e. medical doctors) who, if they offer complementary medicine, usually combine it with conventional medicine.

The acceptance of CAM within mainstream medicine probably depends to a considerable extent on the terminology used. It appears obvious that integration of a CAM approach is only possible when it is based on evidence. Integrative medicine can provide the modern basis for the best possible comprehensive patient care because it combines the strengths of both health care systems (Willich 2009). However, one must be aware that the term 'integrative medicine' is often misused, for example when complementary medicine is offered on limited evidence and/or with a limited focus on the whole person. This treatment is therefore not integrative medicine as defined above and the term complementary would fit better. Overall the term 'complementary and integrative medicine' would, in our opinion, be the most comprehensive and would best reflect the reality in usual care.

In the title and throughout this book we decided to use the term 'complementary medicine' (and, as we mainly deal with treatment evaluation, 'complementary therapies'). In the subtitle we included the term integrative medicine. This might be somewhat arbitrary but it reflects a) our opinion that most of these therapies can be used together with conventional medicine, and b) our optimism that

1

good research could contribute to bringing evidence-based beneficial aspects or interventions from the area of complementary medicine into an integrated medicine.

1.2 The science behind clinical medicine

1.2.1 Major areas of research

Research can be defined as the systematic gathering of data, information and facts for the advancement of scientific knowledge. Following an idealized positivistic view prevailing in biomedicine and natural sciences, scientific knowledge should be unlimited by time and space, i.e. it should consist of facts which apply always and everywhere (although this ideal often seems unrealistic and inadequate for health care research). Basic research in medicine aims to understand the human organism and the mechanisms of disease and it aims to establish the basis for the development of interventions. It encompasses a variety of different disciplines such as molecular biology, biochemistry, physiology and anatomy (➤ Fig. 1.1).

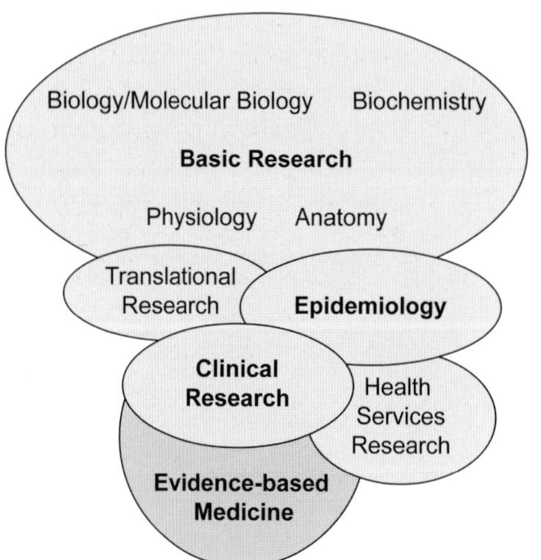

Fig. 1.1 Major areas of research

Clinical research is research on patients or persons at risk dealing with diagnosis, etiology, prevention and treatment of disease as well as maintenance of health.
Clinical research is related to, but not to the same as, epidemiology. The latter discipline studies the causes, distribution, and control of disease in populations. The boundaries between clinical research and epidemiology are not clear-cut, but in general clinical research – albeit usually performed in groups of individuals – focuses on issues directly related to health care interventions and establishes knowledge that can be applied to individual patients, while epidemiology focuses more on observations of groups of people. The area of overlap between clinical research and epidemiology is sometimes called clinical epidemiology. The term 'translational' research has become fashionable in recent years. It indicates the increased effort to link basic and clinical research closely in order to allow a faster transition from development to practice.

It is often forgotten that there is a much broader array of disciplines that is necessary to put biomedical research into context. For example, kybernetics or physics are relevant to basic research. Clinical research should be linked to psychology or social sciences. All this is embedded in epistemological models. The prevailing positivist view in natural sciences has important limitations and has been criticized by different groups including proponents of complementary medicine. We do not feel competent to summarize this discussion here. However we try to reflect broader views when discussing the available research methods with their strengths and limitations even though our book follows mainly a biomedical approach.

Interpreting the facts (hopefully independent of time and space) uncovered by scientific inquiry into clinical practice is a further challenge. Health services research investigates how interventions work within the day to day realities of health care systems, how structures and processes influence outcomes, and whether an innovation is truly cost-effective within a given health system.

1.2.2 Topics in clinical research

When patients seek help from a health care professional they usually present with specific symptoms and signs. Because of their constitution and their behaviour they may have an increased risk of suffering from certain diseases. By taking a case history and doing appropriate examinations the health care professional tries to establish a diagnosis according to the framework of his/her discipline. Implicitly a prognosis is made for the condition without treatment, and, if appropriate, a treatment will be chosen.

For each step in this process, research may contribute important background information (➢ Fig. 1.2). Clinical studies are but systematic attempts to answer questions relevant to health care. Questions for clinical research studies should be operational, that means they should be concise and answerable. Usually answers to clinical research questions are based on some kind of quantitative measurement. Depending on the element of interest in the clinical process and what we exactly want to know about it, a different study design needs to be chosen. For example, if we want to find out how often back pain patients also suffer from major depression we could do a so-called cross-sectional study where back pain sufferers are asked about symptoms of depression. In order to find out whether patients who suffer from low back pain over a longer period of time are more likely to get depression, or in order to gain information on prognosis we may need prospective cohort studies in which a group of patients is followed over a longer period of time. If we want to know whether x-ray examinations are helpful for the diagnosis of non-specific low-back pain we need a diagnostic study. And in order to assess whether a treatment option is effective and safe we would probably look first for evidence from randomized trials or from a systematic review of such trials.

1.2.3 Evidence-based medicine

The current ideal of how science should be incorporated into the health care of individual patients is evidence-based medicine (EBM).

> "Evidence based medicine is defined as the conscientious, explicit, and judicious use of current best scientific evidence in making decisions about the care of individual patients. The practice of evidence based medicine means integrating individual clinical expertise with the best available external clinical evidence from systematic research." (Sackett et al., 1996)
> While this definition applies to the level of the individual health care provider and patient, the term evidence-based medicine is increasingly used also for making decisions for whole health care systems based on evidence from clinical studies.

1.3 Why do we need research on complementary therapies?

Each day a health care provider seeing patients has to make countless decisions. If, for example the practitioner wants to treat Mr. Miller, a 38-year man with chronic low back pain, with acupuncture and

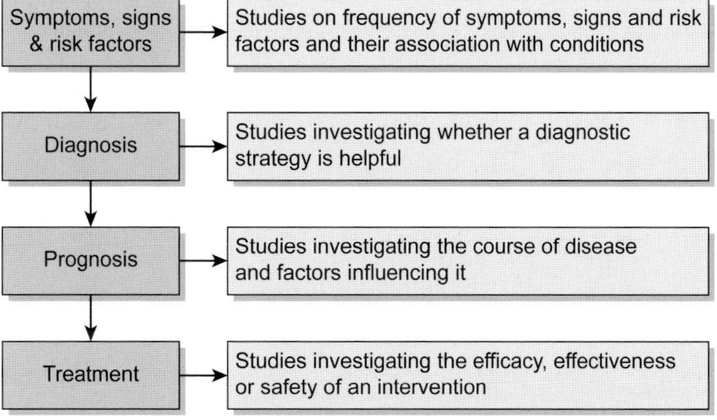

Fig. 1.2 Main steps in the care of individual patients and related studies

1

hypnosis this decision is typically based on a variety of factors:
- individual experience (the provider has seen similar patients who improved with this therapy),
- theoretical considerations (based on the therapy's concept, it makes sense to use this particular therapy in this patient),
- expectations and preferences of the patient (the patient wants or at least accepts this therapy),
- aspects such as feasibility (the provider can do it with this patient)
- economical considerations (the provider can earn a living providing the therapy).

Where does research enter in here?

Many providers have busy clinics and say that patients are voting with their feet. Why should they embark on the cumbersome route of scientific research which, in the end, might not bring desired results? On the other hand, sceptics consider investment in research in CAM a waste of resources. Why then do we believe that (more) research into complementary therapies is necessary?

We think there are reasons on several different levels:
- There is an **ethical mandate to evaluate the safety and effectiveness of health care interventions**. Any therapy including complementary medicine contributes to the health care market and should thus be assessed. The history of medicine is full of interventions which may have appeared beneficial at one time but after careful evaluation may have turned out to be harmful. A famous example is the excessive use of bloodletting in the past. Even interventions which are, in principle, safe and effective should be evaluated carefully to find the appropriate indications. The herb St John's Wort (Hypericum perforatum) has been used widely for the treatment of depression and related disorders, but it became clear recently that it interacts with other, sometimes life-saving, drugs. Research is crucial here to help decide when St John's Wort should be used and when not.
- It is of **considerable scientific interest to find out whether and how specific complementary therapies work**. From the perspective of natural sciences the theoretical background of most complementary medicine is speculative or implausible, but CAM therapists tend to have specific convictions about elements in their therapy that are crucial for achieving effective treatment. Since the truly characteristic component of the therapy is not known for certain, many trials comparing complementary therapies with sham or placebo interventions could have been conducted under suboptimal conditions. The results have very often been very disappointing for CAM therapists, though reassuring for sceptics. Nevertheless, complementary therapies frequently perform well when compared to usual care, which suggests that other mechanisms are important. There is increasing evidence that some complementary therapies have strong placebo effects. Research into complementary medicine may have a leading role in investigating how such effects may be better used in all types of medicine. Some CAM providers may dislike this reasoning, but it would certainly add to the value of CAM research if it had an additional positive impact on medicine overall.
- **Scientific evidence on complementary therapies is needed to develop evidence-based integrative medicine**.
- **Politicians and other stakeholders need reliable information for making decisions** whether therapies should be licensed, reimbursed, recommended, discouraged or banned. Political decisions cannot, and should not, rely exclusively on scientific evidence. Preferences, cultural acceptability, feasibility and costs are also important for making decisions in any society. Nevertheless, research evidence is *one* crucial component and appropriate evidence should be available.
- Last but not least: research can and should lead to **improvement of clinical care**. Challenging established theories and processes together with developing new ideas can help to improve health care – this applies also to complementary medicine.

To be useful, research into complementary therapies has to be of high quality, avoiding the influence of bias in methods and results, and should primarily reflect the interests of patients and society.

1.4 Is research into complementary therapies special?

1.4.1 Why research into complementary therapies is somewhat different?

Is research into complementary therapies any different from research in conventional medicine? In principle, the answer to this question is clearly: no! Medicine, biology, psychology, and social sciences have developed a large toolkit of study designs to find answers for a huge variety of different questions. If appropriate use is made of the available methods, research into complementary therapies does not need its own methods - in principle. However, in practice, there are some factors which make complementary medicine research slightly different.

The most important single reason for this difference is probably the historical point at which complementary therapies are evaluated.

Consider the process of drug development in conventional medicine. Based on the biochemical and physiological understanding of the mechanisms of a disease, a new substance is developed and tested in cell lines and animals. If the findings are promising and do not indicate any obvious risks, the four consecutive phases of clinical research begin (➢ Fig. 1.3 left):

- In **phase I** safety and pharmacological effects are tested in a small number of healthy volunteers and patients.
- In **phase II** the new drug must be shown to be safe and to have some beneficial effects ("proof of concept"), still in a limited number of patients (usually between 50 and 200). Furthermore, dose-finding is an important aim in phase II.
- The main test of clinical efficacy occurs in **phase III** mostly with placebo-controlled randomized trials. Depending on the condition the number of patients varies between several hundred and several thousand. These trials are the crucial step for licensing.

Only if a significant effect over placebo or non-inferiority to a proven standard treatment is shown is the drug licensed and becomes available on the market.

- After licensing, **phase IV** studies are performed for a variety of reasons, such as detecting rare side effects, establishing cost-effectiveness or marketing by the drug company. Phase IV studies are often very large including usually more than 1,000 patients per study.
- The crucial point is this: the drug is only available *after* it has been licensed and the evaluation has been considered successful. Non-drug interventions in conventional medicine often do not undergo similar systematic testing, though there is commonly some scientific evaluation *before* they become widely available.

In complementary medicine the situation is very often the other way round. Most complementary treatments only become scientifically evaluated *after* their use has become so widespread that they cannot be ignored any longer. This has important implications:

- Providers have already treated many patients and are convinced that their treatments are beneficial. So providers are often reluctant to agree that their patients may be randomized to treatment and placebo, respectively.
- If a treatment has been available over a long period of time and from large numbers of providers, there

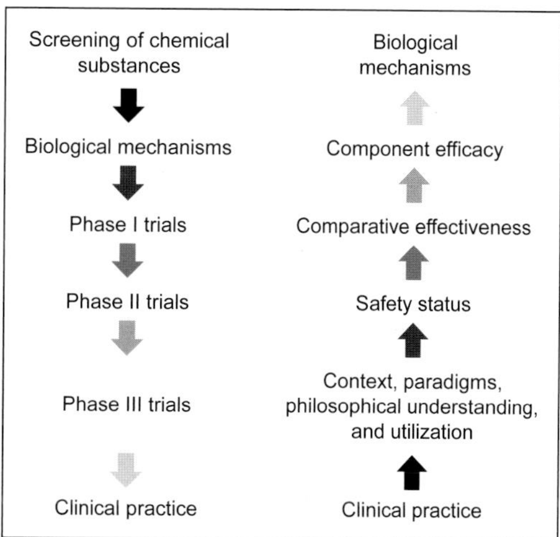

Fig. 1.3 Phases in drug research vs. phases in complementary medicine research adapted from Fønnebø et al. (2007)

is likely to be some diversification, i.e. different providers apply the therapy in a slightly, or sometimes very, different manner. The question then arises whether the results of a study done in one style can be extrapolated to another style.
- Patients treated with complementary medicine often actively choose "their" therapy and develop strong preferences or have strong beliefs. However results from studies done in such subjects may not apply to patients not actively seeking complementary medicine. And if a study is done in the latter group, it is at least questionable whether it is relevant to "believers".
- Finally, if an experimental study finds a negative result, will CAM providers and patients accept "statistical findings" which contradict their direct personal experience? A drug which does not show efficacy in phase III never becomes available, but can health authorities ban a widely practised complementary therapy if a randomized trial is negative?

1.4.2 Strategic approaches to research into complementary medicine

Cardini et al. (2006) and Fønnebø et al. (2007) have proposed that the phases of research may be reversed for complementary medicine (➢ Fig. 1.3 right):
- Researchers should first observe clinical practice to find out
  - which therapies are widely used,
  - how they are used,
  - by whom they are used, and
  - why they are used.
- As a next step, the evaluation of safety is crucial because if an intervention is truly harmful it should be banned.
- An investigation of how the therapy compares to other treatments should follow.
- Only if there is a positive result from the preceding steps would it be of interest to find out which components of the therapy are relevant to its clinical effect and investigate the therapy's theory.

However, in most cases the evaluation of a complementary therapy will not be strictly sequential, but single studies will address a specific aspect depending on priorities, resources, interests and feasibility. Some studies will assess efficacy over placebo or effectiveness over routine care, other trials will investigate preferences, relevance, safety or mechanisms and so on. If evidence from several levels accumulates, a meaningful mosaic may emerge. Walach et al. (2006) have argued that a circular approach would be the most appropriate way to evaluate complex complementary treatments. Such a circular approach seems applicable to complementary medicine research in a broad way. Based on what is available so far, one decides which aspects are most relevant at the next level. The box below gives an example of the questions currently discussed in relation to a medicinal herb widely used as antidepressant (St John's Wort).

- How widespread is the use of St John's Wort extracts for treatment of depressive disorders?
- Who prescribes St John's Wort extracts?
- Which patients buy them of their own accord?
- Why are they using St John's Wort instead of proven standard antidepressants?
- How does availability and use vary between different countries?
- Are St. John's Wort extracts more effective than placebo and equally effective as standard antidepressants?
- Do they have fewer side effects?
- Can they be taken with other drugs?
- Is there pharmacological evidence for their antidepressant effects from laboratory research?
- Which components are contributing to these effects?
- Are the different products on the market pharmacologically comparable and equally effective?

1.4.3 Why it is difficult to realize strategic approaches?

Systematic strategic approaches would be of great importance but several factors do not make them very easy:
- The number of interventions in complementary medicine and conditions treated is huge,
- the research infrastructure in CAM settings is still quite small, and
- funding – with a few exceptions – is minimal.

It might sound impressive if *several million* euros or dollars are spent on "investigating the effectiveness of complementary medicine", but getting one single new drug from development to licensing costs *several hundred millions.* Expecting that a few studies will provide all answers is therefore completely unrealistic.

Finally, the aim of research in complementary medicine is often problematic. In conventional medicine, the ultimate goal of research is (or at least, should be) improvement of patient care. However the goal of research in complementary medicine seems very often to be to prove to the world that your view is correct (i.e. that your therapy is effective if you are a convinced provider, or that it is rubbish if you are a skeptic).

Prior beliefs seem to be particularly strong in the discussion of complementary therapies and any study will be criticized, regardless of its results.

Therefore, the self-critical attitude crucial to any good research is also very important in complementary medicine research.

Given the multiplicity of unresolved questions, a large variety of research is required in the area of complementary medicine. However, since the resources are limited and the area so vast, it is necessary to set priorities. This is very difficult. For example, for several years clinical trials evaluating the efficacy of widely used treatments were the top priority of NCCAM. While such studies remain a focus of its funding, in its strategic plan for the years 2005 to 2009 (www.nccam.nih.gov) the NCCAM planned to invest more money in "preliminary studies" before investing in large clinical trials. For example, NCCAM favoured studies on quality control of a herbal product, optimal doses, or appropriate subject populations.

In some areas of complementary medicine basic research on mechanisms is of utmost importance. For example, if basic research could come up with a scientifically plausible theory of a mechanism of action for homeopathy, the impact would be much more profound than new clinical trials on effectiveness. Thus one could argue that investing in research on potential mechanisms should be a top priority of research into homeopathy. However, if such research does not produce convincing findings, what does this mean? Does it tell us whether homeopathy really helps patients, whether its costs should be reimbursed or whether it should be banned? In conclusion, basic research is crucial but it should not be the only focus in the research of a complementary therapy.

In conclusion, there can be little doubt that research on effectiveness and safety must and will remain one main focus for most complementary therapies.

1.5 Aims, target audience and structure of this book

This book aims to provide the necessary knowledge to understand and produce high quality clinical research on effectiveness and efficacy of complementary medicine interventions.

The primary target audience of this book is individuals who are interested in becoming actively involved in complementary medicine research.

➢ Chapters 2 and 3 provide basic knowledge on the main steps that must be understood before doing a study – study design and statistics. The core ➢ chapters 4 to 7 aim to help a researcher to successfully plan, manage, analyse and publish a clinical study of a CAM treatment. Each chapter contains detailed, practical and step-by-step descriptions of what to do when and how. In these chapters we commonly also include three case studies as practical examples – one is an uncontrolled observational study, one a randomized double-blind placebo-controlled trial and one a pragmatic randomized trial comparing three groups. Throughout the chapters, they grow into true full research studies whose final abstracts can be found in the ➢ appendix. ➢ Chapters 8 to 10 provide introductions to research methods (surveys, qualitative research, health economics, single case studies). These help researchers to put the results of their clinical study into a broader context. In the final chapter (➢ Ch. 11) we briefly introduce methods for research on prevalence, diagnosis and etiology.

REFERENCES

Cardini F, Wade C, Regalia AL, Gui S, Li W, Raschetti R, Kronenberg F. Clinical research in traditional medicine: priorities and methods. Complement Ther Med 2006;14:282–287.

Dobos G. Integrative Medicine – Medicine of the future or ‚Old Wine in New Skins'? Eur J Integrat Med 2009;1:109–115.

Fletcher RW, Fletcher SW. Clinical epidemiology. The essentials. 4th edition. Philadelphia: Lippincott, Williams & Wilkins, 2005.

Fønnebø V, Grimsgaard S, Walach H, Ritenbaugh C, Norheim AJ, MacPherson H, Lewith G, Launsø L, Koithan M, Falkenberg T, Boon H, Aickin M. Researching complementary and alternative treatments – the gatekeepers are not at home. BMC Med Res Methodol. 2007; 7:7.

Haynes RB, Sackett DL, Guyatt GH, Tugwell P. Clinical epidemiology. How to do clinical practice research. 3rd edition. Philadelphia: Lippincott, Williams & Wilkins, 2005.

Hulley SB, Cummings SR, Browner WS, Grady DG, Newman TB. Designing clinical research. 3rd edition. Philadelphia: Lippincott, Williams & Wilkins, 2007.

Katz MH. Study design and statistical analysis. A practical guide for clinicians. Cambridge: Cambridge University Press, 2007.

Recommend textbooks on the whole spectrum of clinical research methods.

Sackett DL, Rosenberg WM, Gray JA, Haynes RB, Richardson WS. Evidence based medicine: what it is and what it isn't. BMJ 1996;312:71–72.

Walach H, Falkenberg T, Fønnebø V, Lewith G, Jonas WB. Circular instead of hierarchical: methodological principles for the evaluation of complex interventions. BMC Med Res Methodol 2006;6:29.

Willich SN. Editorial. Eur J Integrat Med 2009;1:163–164.

I Theory – Things you should know before embarking on a clinical study

The first part of this book summarizes what you should know before starting a clinical study yourself: we provide introductions to (i) study design for research on efficacy and effectiveness (➤ Ch. 2) and to (ii) statistics (➤ Ch. 3)

CHAPTER 2 Basic study design

2.1 When is a treatment effective?

2.1.1 Why do we need control or comparison groups?

When is a treatment effective? The most basic answer to this question is, when a patient is better off with the treatment than without. So how do studies need to be done to answer this question? One could simply think of studies observing a group of patients and measuring how patients are before and after the treatment. Some people say that if patients are better after treatment this is evidence that the treatment worked. However this reasoning is too simplistic. Imagine a study in which 50 people suffering from a common cold receive a herbal remedy. After 7 days the participants have on average fewer cold symptoms than before treatment (➢ Fig. 2.1). Does this truly mean that the treatment was effective? Clearly not, as we do not know **the natural course of disease** in these patients. In other words, how would these individuals have done without treatment?

Imagine now that you have a group of 10 patients suffering from advanced cancer with very poor prognosis. If you had a treatment that completely cured all these patients you could be rather sure that it was highly effective. From all that you know about advanced cancer (that is, if you are certain about the evidence that these patients have a very poor prognosis) you would predict that cure without treatment – or even with the treatments presently available – would be highly unlikely. You have a virtual comparison group in mind with a clear idea how these patients would have done without the treatment. In most cases, however, the effects of treatments are less dramatic and you need a concurrent control or comparison, as in the example of the herbal remedy for colds (➢ Fig. 2.2). If you have a control group, you compare the outcome in the treatment and control groups and the difference between these two is the treatment effect – not the difference in each group before and after treatment! In this way you control for the natural course of the disease as well as for other problems described below.

Some people argue that CAM treatments are often used in chronically ill individuals in whom spontaneous improvement is unlikely. However, the severity of complaints of most chronic conditions varies considerably over time. This is termed **spontaneous fluctuation of symptoms** (which is nothing other than a specific type of natural course of the disease). Patients are much more likely to seek treatment in phases during which complaints are severe or increasing than in phases in which they feel relatively well. Therefore, control groups are usually also needed in studies of chronically ill patients.

Control groups also take account of another problem relevant to clinical studies: regression to the mean.

> Regression to the mean is the statistical phenomenon whereby individuals with extreme values on a given measure for one observation will, for purely statistical reasons, probably give less extreme measurements on other occasions when they are observed.

Imagine you have a sample of 1,000 healthy individuals whose average systolic blood pressure over 6 months is about 120 mmHg. You measure blood pressure in these individuals once and then include all, let's say 50, "patients" with a value over 140 mmHg into a study. You give them a drug and after four weeks the average blood pressure is 120 mmHg. It should be obvious that you cannot attribute this improvement to the drug (or only to the drug) as it is likely that most of these non-hypertensive individuals would have a more normal result at a second measurement anyway. While nobody would set up

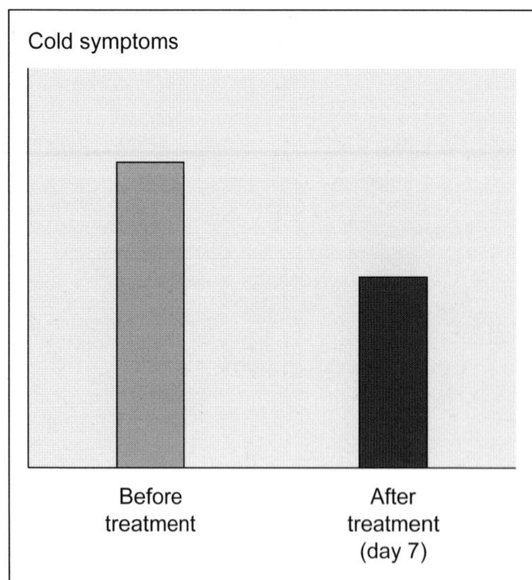

Fig. 2.1 Study without a control group investigating the intensity of symptoms in a group of patients with a common cold

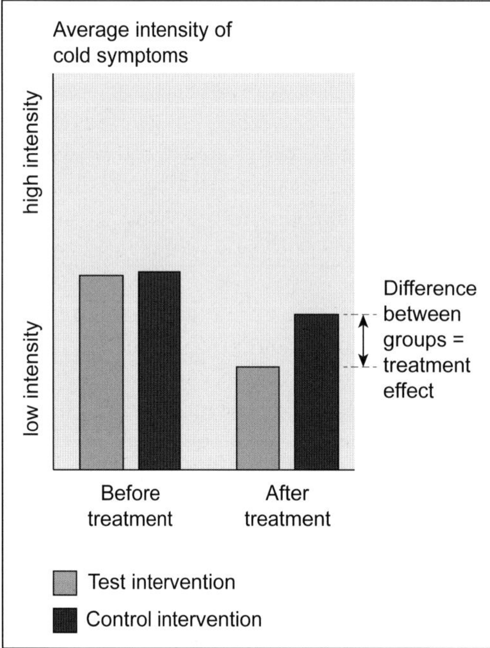

Fig. 2.2 Study with a control group investigating the intensity of symptoms in a group of patients with a common cold

such a study, the problem is to some extent very real in clinical trials.

For example, many studies on chronic low back pain include only patients who report a minimum pain level such as 40 mm on a 100 mm visual analogue scale (= VAS, a line with ends labelled for example 'no pain' and 'extreme pain', on which patients are asked to indicate the intensity of their complaints with a mark). It makes no sense to include patients who only have little pain, because there is not much room for improvement. However the problem associated with this practice is that, because symptoms of many conditions vary over time, you are likely to get at least some regression to the mean. Even if the average pain of the patients checked for inclusion in your studies is above 40 mm, some of them will have had less pain in the weeks before study inclusion, just by chance. These patients are not included into the study (➤ Fig. 2.3). If you observe the included patients for several weeks you would expect that the mean of pain ratings will decrease.

In summary, control or comparison groups are fundamental for evaluating whether a treatment is effective as they show changes due to the natural course of diseases, spontaneous fluctuations and regression to the mean. The treatment effect is the difference of the outcome in the treatment group versus the control group, and not the difference of before and after treatment in each group.

2.1.2 Types of controls and comparisons

You can show the effectiveness of your treatment in a number of ways (➤ Table 2.1) and the choice of your control or comparison will depend on the question you want to answer. The most basic question is whether your treatment is superior to doing nothing. However, in many situations it is unethical to leave patients untreated. This means that you may want to show at least that adding your treatment to usual or standard care results in an additional benefit. As we will see below, studies comparing treatment with no treatment or investigating a treatment as an addition to usual or standard care suffer from several problems, and it is impossible to tell whether any additional effects are due to specific or non-specific elements of the treatment. Therefore, one would also like to see evidence that a treatment is better than placebo.

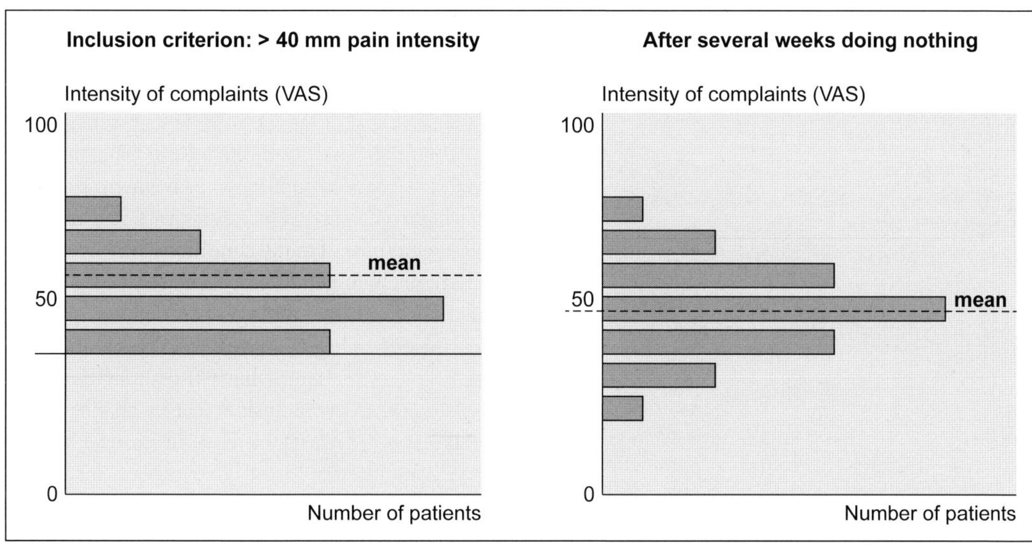

Fig. 2.3 Example of regression to the mean – since only patients with a pain score > 40 on a 100 mm visual analogue scale are included and because it is likely that later measurements will include lower values due to normal pain fluctuations, the mean of observations will decrease

Table 2.1 Ways to show that a treatment is effective

Question	Type of effect assessed	What you are looking for
Is my treatment better than doing nothing?	Total (non-specific and specific) effect	Superiority
Is my treatment a useful addition to basic or standard care?	Total (non-specific and specific) effect (as addition)	Superiority
Is my treatment better than a placebo?	Specific effect	Superiority
Is my treatment better than another (effective) treatment	Comparison of total effects (Comparative effect)	Superiority
Is my treatment at least as good as another (effective) treatment	Comparison of total effects (Comparative effect)	Non-inferiority
Is my treatment as good as another (effective) treatment	Comparison of total effects (Comparative effect)	Equivalence

If you have discovered a new treatment alternative for a life-threatening condition for which a proven treatment is available, a comparison with no treatment or placebo is ethically not acceptable. As your treatment is an alternative to the old standard treatment and not an addition you have to show that it is at least not inferior to, or as good as (equivalent), the proven standard. The difference between the terms non-inferiority (which does not rule out that your treatment is better) and equivalence will be explained further in ➢ Ch. 3. Preferably you would, however, want to show that your treatment is better (superior) than the proven standard.

Comparisons with available standard treatments are not just relevant to new interventions. In general, the question of how one approach for managing a disease compares to the results of other approaches is usually the most realistic and important one for routine care. The relevance of such **comparative effectiveness research** is also shown by the U.S. administration's decision to spend more than 1 billion USD for this purpose in the years 2009 to 2011 (Convay and Glancy 2009).

Preferably you will have an assortment of studies showing evidence of effects over no treatment or over usual care only, as well as over placebo, or else you will have studies showing at least non-inferiority to established standard treatment.

The term **control group** implies that you have this group controlling for a number of potential influences. In clinical research it is typically used when a comparison is made with groups receiving placebo, no treatment or usual care only. In basic research, controlled often means that you also try to standardize as many other variables (procedures, temperature, day time etc.) as possible. The term **comparison group** is broader and more neutral. In clinical research it is used more frequently if the alternative option is an active treatment. As the distinction between the two terms is rather vague we will use them as synonyms in the following text.

2.1.3 Specific and non-specific effects

From the perspective of natural sciences most CAM treatments have little plausibility. For materialist scientists, life energy and its flow through meridians is at best an imaginary concept, and the idea that highly potentized homeopathic remedies containing practically nothing but milk sugar or alcohol can have any direct effect on the human body is implausible. Therefore, almost inevitably, the question arises whether any clinical effects observed for CAM therapies are anything more than placebo effects. The traditional concept of specific and non-specific (= placebo) effects has been developed mainly with regards to drugs, but is applied to non-drug interventions too. It is commonly assumed that the total therapeutic effect of a drug intervention consists of both specific and non-specific effects. The specific effects are those which are due to the active ingredient while the non-specific (or placebo) effects are due to psychological or psychophysiological effects associated with the act of treatment.

The traditional concept of specific and non-specific effects seems straightforward, but it has severe drawbacks. A major problem is that one has to define what is specific about an intervention and what nonspecific. In the case of drugs this is straightforward. The active substance has to make a difference. We would not accept an expensive new drug if it only worked by symbolic means. However, if the mechanism of action is completely unclear, or if the treatment under investigation is a complex intervention, then it becomes difficult to separate specific and non-specific components. Psychotherapy is a good (non-CAM) example: there are several different types of psychotherapy. Based on theoretical considerations, proponents of a particular method have made claims about what makes their method different from (and better than) other methods. Trials which tried to investigate the specific contributions of these characteristic components quite often did not find any effects over "non-specific" comparator treatments. But these comparator treatments could not be considered inert, and the theoretical considerations defining specific and non-specific

In the traditional concept "a placebo is defined as any therapy or component of therapy used for its nonspecific, psychological, or psychophysiological effect, or that is used for its presumed specific effect, but is without specific activity for the condition being treated. [...] A placebo, when used as a control in experimental studies, is defined as a substance or procedure that is without specific activity for the condition being treated." (Shapiro and Morris 1978)
According to this concept, a three-armed trial with the intervention of interest, a placebo intervention and a no treatment control can quantify specific and non-specific effects of a treatment (➤ Fig. 2.4).

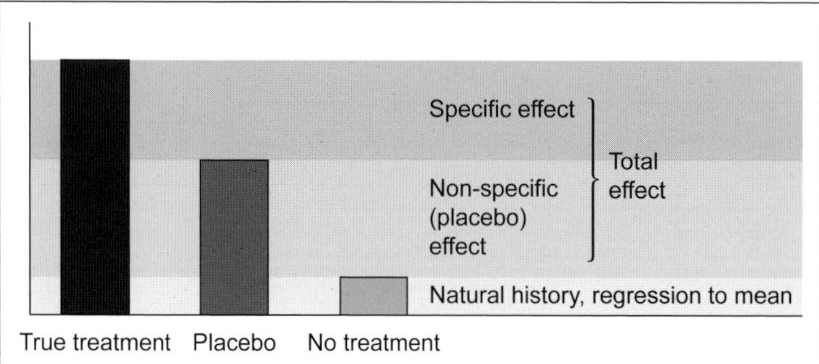

Fig. 2.4 The traditional concept of non-specific (placebo) and specific effects

components might have been wrong. Can we really consider these non-specific comparator treatments as placebos? For many CAM treatments the situation is to some extent similar, and probably even worse. Many assumptions regarding mechanisms for CAM therapies are highly speculative. Most homeopaths assume that their remedies retain specific information despite being chemically indistinguishable from the diluent. Many acupuncturists are convinced that the most important aspects of their treatment are skin penetration, correct point selection and appropriate method of stimulation. Available research suggests that these (simple, mechanistic) theories are at least incomplete or maybe even simply wrong. Acupuncture points may have some specific effects but recent research strongly suggests that psychophysiological effects play an important role, too. These problems are partly reflected by the fact that, in trials of non-drug treatments, control interventions without the presumed specific component are often called **sham treatment** instead of placebo. However, interpreting sham acupuncture interventions as equivalent to giving a placebo pill is probably not correct.

Another major problem with the traditional placebo concept is that it is extremely vague about how placebo effects can occur. If a placebo does not cause any effects by itself how can it have psychophysiological effects?

The term '**meaning response**' has been proposed as an alternative to the term placebo effect (Moerman and Jonas 2002). According to this concept, the placebo intervention only completes an interaction in a healing environment by giving it a meaning. Depending on the meaning of the whole interaction positive (placebo), negative (nocebo) or no effect occur. Other authors have proposed the term **'context effect'** (di Blasi et al. 2001) indicating that a variety of context factors such as expectations, experiences, attitudes, relationship, setting, etc. shape the meaning of an intervention and modify the size of potential responses of an individual.

Neurophysiological and clinical research on placebo effects has shown that expectations, conditioning, learning, or anxiety reduction are important pathways for triggering the psychophysiological processes that are the basis of placebo effects. Through these pathways placebo stimuli can have marked effects on the brain all of which are obviously context-dependent (Benedetti 2008, comprehensive review). It might be that many CAM treatments (as well as symbolically powerful conventional treatments such as surgery) are associated with particularly strong meaning or context effects.

In summary, placebo controls are a crucial tool for investigating which part of the total clinical effect of an intervention is due to those components which are considered specific or characteristic according to the postulated theory. However, there are reasons to believe that theories of mechanisms in CAM are often incomplete or even wrong, and that the size of placebo effects depends of the meaning and context of and interventions. This complicates the *clinical* interpretation of placebo-controlled clinical trials

2.2 Bias – threats to internal validity

The inclusion of a control or comparison group allows us to compare the outcomes of these patients with those of the patients receiving the intervention of interest. The difference between the groups is the fundamental result of a study. However, the difference can be distorted by bias.

Bias is the "systematic distortion of the estimated intervention effect away from the 'truth', caused by inadequacies in the design, conduct, or analysis of a trial."
"A study which is not biased has high internal validity. Internal validity means the extent to which the design and conduct of a study eliminate the possibility of bias." (www.consort-statement.org/resources/glossary)

2.2.1 Prognostic and baseline differences between groups – why randomization is so desirable

One straightforward way to compare, for example, the effectiveness of homeopathy and conventional medicine in treating patients with sinusitis would be to include patients meeting defined inclusion criteria treated by homeopathic and conventional physicians. This would be a realistic reflection of what actually happens in the real world, and, in fact, such a study has been done (Weber et al., 2000).

While this set-up may reflect real life, it is almost impossible to tell from its results which treatment is more effective, since observed outcome differences between groups may arise from different prognoses due to confounding factors. **Confounding** means that there are differences between the comparison groups, apart from the planned interventions, which have an impact on the outcomes observed.

A famous example of the influence of confounding and selection bias was the belief in the 1990s that hormone replacement therapy protects women from myocardial infarction. Based on a plausible rationale and data from observational studies comparing rates of myocardial infarction among women taking hormone replacement therapy and those who did not, this therapy was recommended by many physicians and researchers. This recommendation was only stopped when a large randomized controlled showed that there was actually a slightly harmful effect of hormone replacement therapy. The lower incidence of myocardial infarction among women taking hormones in the observational studies was at least partly due to the fact that women with higher socio-economic status (which is clearly associated with a lower risk of myocardial infarction) were more likely to receive hormone replacement therapy.

In the homeopathic sinusitis study, patients with more acute symptoms were more often treated by conventional physicians, while patients with more recurrent or chronic problems more often went to a homeopath. According to methodological language the 'true' difference was distorted by 'selection bias' (which is one type of confounding). In other words it is a race in which runners start from different positions. Although there are adjustment methods to account for prognostic or baseline differences, e.g. by matching patients with similar prognostic indicators or by complex statistical analyses (see below), adjustment methods should only be the second choice.

Randomization (syn. random allocation or random assignment) is the best method to ensure a fair comparison and avoid selection bias (➤ Fig. 2.5).

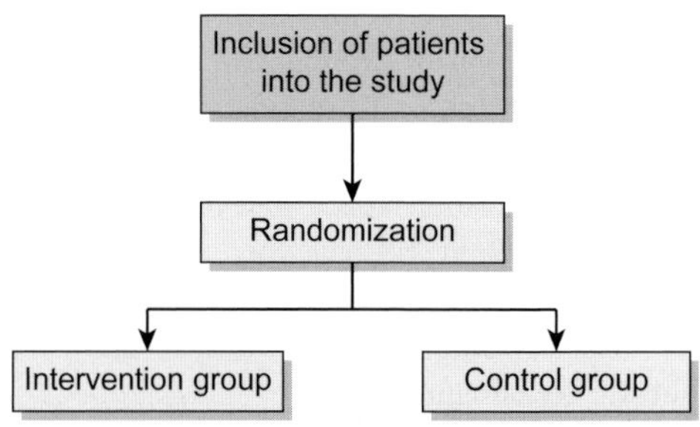

Fig. 2.5 Randomization – Patients are first included in a trial and then allocated in a type of lottery to the intervention and the control group

Randomization means that the decision whether a patient becomes allocated to the treatment group or the control group is not made by patient, physician or anyone else, but is random and thus unpredictable.
Randomization is clearly not what patients or providers would like to do in normal practice, but is the best way to find out whether any differences in clinical outcomes are due to the treatment applied.

It has to be kept in mind that randomization does not always generate groups which are comparable for all baseline characteristics. Particularly if studies are small, it can easily happen that there are baseline differences between groups just by chance. If baseline differences occur in spite of randomization, statisticians try to "adjust" for them in complex statistical analyses. These important methods will briefly be discussed in the statistics section. They are routinely used in epidemiological research where it is often impossible to randomize patients, for example, to find out whether increases in leukaemia rates in children living close to nuclear power plants are truly due to the proximity of the plant or to other factors.

Adjustment methods can and should also be used in nonrandomized comparisons of treatments (➤ Ch. 3.6). However, it is only possible to adjust for those factors which have been actually measured. As we often do not know exactly what predicts an outcome in a patient it is likely that we miss important factors. This may also be the case in a randomized comparison, but randomization also distributes non-measured factors with equal chance to the groups. So unless randomization fails by chance, groups are similar both in respect to measured and unmeasured factors at baseline.

2.2.2 Differences between groups after treatment has started – why blinding is so desirable

Even if randomization has created groups which are well comparable at baseline there are still many ways in which the findings of a trial can be biased. There may be some differences in how groups are handled after baseline apart from the treatment under test. Patients randomized to a no treatment group may be disappointed and therefore rate subjective outcome scales in a different manner, or may use more effective co-interventions. Physicians may expect less improvement in such patients and rate symptoms more pessimistically. On the other hand, in some instances physicians may prescribe other, more effective, non-study interventions to compensate the perceived lack of treatment or to improve burdening symptoms. If therapists have direct financial interest in a treatment or simply want to prove that they are right they may even deliberately bias assessments.

The major tool for minimizing bias during a study after allocation to groups is blinding (also called masking). Whenever possible treatment providers, patients and, if applicable, outcome assessors should be unaware of individual group allocation (➤ Fig. 2.6).
Of course, in comparisons with no treatment, or with two clearly distinguishable treatments, patients and providers cannot be blinded. Therefore, such comparisons often have limited internal validity, particularly if all relevant outcomes are subjective. Sometimes it is possible to blind outcome assessment by having this done by an independent person unaware of who received what.

It has to be kept in mind that, even if investigators do their best to blind patients, providers or other trial participants may find out the allocation status of an individual. This is called **unblinding**. Unblinding can happen due to characteristic side effects of a treatment, due to a different appearance of a treatment, or even because a treatment may show distinct (beneficial) effects. Thus bias may be introduced even in trials described as blind.

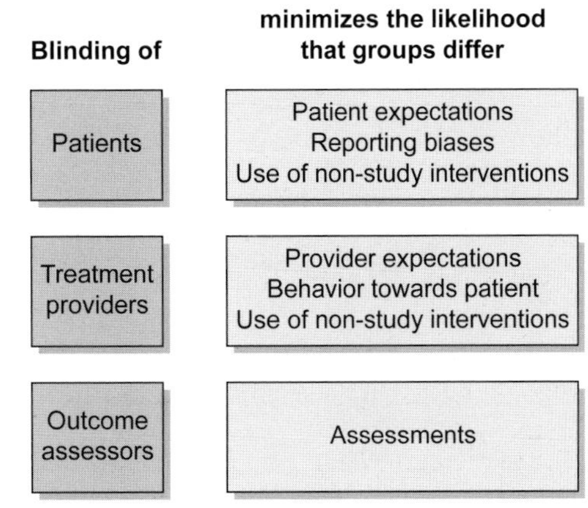

Fig. 2.6 Blinding of key individuals in controlled trials and its function

2.2.3 Attrition

A major problem in most studies with longer observation periods is that some patients included in the study drop out prematurely or do not follow the study protocol.

The terms attrition, drop-out, withdrawal or loss to follow-up are used to indicate that not all participants included in a study complete it.
Attrition is used as a general term to describe this issue. Drop-out usually means that a patient actively leaves a study, withdrawal is often used in a similar manner but can also indicate that the investigators excluded an individual. Loss to follow-up usually indicates that patients did not show up for scheduled examinations. However, the delineation between these terms is vague.

If, for example, only 60 % of the patients included in a study of acupuncture for chronic low back pain are available for follow-up, it is difficult or even impossible to interpret the data. The outcome of patients remaining in the study may differ considerably from those dropping out (➤ Fig. 2.7). Those drop-outs may have experienced worsening of symptoms more often (or, possibly, cure more often), they may have experienced more severe side effects, been unsatisfied etc. The best method to prevent bias due to attrition is to keep it as low as possible, for example, by limiting the frequency and duration of follow-up

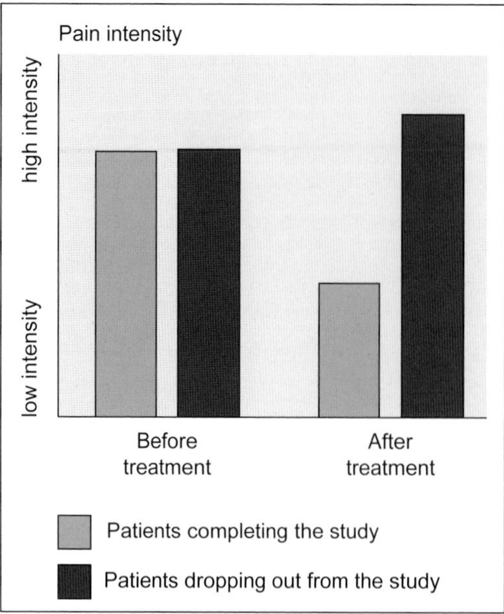

Fig. 2.7 Example of how the selective drop-out of patients with bad outcomes leads to an overestimation of changes over time

visits, or by performing telephone interviews to gather at least some key data.

It is almost impossible to interpret studies without a control group if drop-out rates are high, but the situation is not much better in studies with a control group, particularly if the number or reasons for drop-outs differ between groups.

As some degree of attrition is almost inevitable in studies with longer observation periods, it is necessary that the statistical analysis takes it into account. Whenever possible the analysis should include all patients which were randomized or chose a treatment. This is called intention to treat analysis. If the attrition rate is not too high there are also methods which impute missing data (➢ Ch. 3).

2.2.4 Bias during analysis and reporting

Bias may be introduced not only at allocation and while the study is performed, but also when it is analyzed and reported. For example, patients with "implausible" (undesired) findings may be excluded from the analysis. If the predefined main outcome does not yield the expected result, another outcome may be declared as main outcome measure during or after running the study. While such actions are clear misconduct, there is plenty of evidence of such bias in the medical literature (McGauran et al. 2010). The remedy for inappropriate exclusion of patients from the analysis is the above-mentioned intention to treat analysis. To reduce the likelihood that studies with undesired outcomes disappear into filing-cabinet drawers or that main outcomes are re-defined, randomized clinical trials are now routinely registered in web-based clinical trial registries. Another solution is to publish the study protocol in a journal before a study is started or early during the study.

2.3 Clinical studies and the real world – external validity

2.3.1 The need for balancing internal and external validity

After reading section 2.1.3 you may have got the impression that we believe all clinical studies evaluating a therapy should be randomized, blinded trials with an intention to treat analysis because such studies have high internal validity and a low risk of bias. But it's not that simple. Clinical studies should be both scientific and helpful for actual decision making. This is not an easy task. The scientist would like to have the study controlled and as internally valid as possible in order to be sure that any difference observed between the outcomes of the intervention and the control group is only due to the "independent variable" (the difference in the intervention). Therefore preference is given to the inclusion of a homogeneous group of patients who are compliant and who do not have any relevant co-morbidity in a randomized, blinded trial with clearly defined and standardized interventions. However, does information from such a trial truly inform the practitioner who cares for highly heterogeneous individuals with variable co-morbidity and compliance to treatment? Therefore, when planning and doing clinical studies, compromises have to be made balancing internal and external validity, efficacy and effectiveness, and explanatory or pragmatic approaches.

External validity is the extent to which the results of a trial provides a correct basis for generalizations to other circumstances (www.consort-statement.org/resources/glossary). **Efficacy** refers to 'the extent to which a specific intervention is beneficial under ideal conditions'. **Effectiveness** is a 'measure of the extent to which a specific intervention when deployed in the field in routine circumstances does what it is intended to do for a specific population' (Last et al. 2001).
Trials designed to help choose between different options for care are called **pragmatic**. Trials designed to test causal research hypotheses – for example, that an intervention causes a particular biological change – are called **explanatory** (Schwartz and Lelouch 1967).

These concepts and terms form a complex and flexible framework in which clinical studies can reasonably well be classified. Note that the adjective 'effective' is used here (and throughout this book) both in relation to efficacy and effectiveness trials because the word 'efficacious' is uncommon. The term trial is used only for randomized studies; so keep in mind that pragmatic *trials* are always randomized. A non-randomized, pragmatic comparative effectiveness study is not considered a trial.

➢ Table 2.2 summarizes two very different randomized trials investigating the effects of acupuncture for headache. In a small Swedish acupuncture trial, M. Linde et al. (2005) investigated in one specialized migraine clinic whether skin penetration makes a significant difference in women with menstrually related migraine. Patients were highly selected and the true acupuncture intervention was highly standardized. As sham intervention, non-penetrating acupuncture needles were applied at exactly the same points as in the true treatment group. As some points were on the head all patients had to wear a special cap. The authors tried very hard to make the true and the sham acupuncture intervention as indistinguishable as possible, in order to reduce the likelihood of bias and to maximise internal validity. If this trial had found a difference in the clinical outcomes between the groups (it did not) this would have been evidence for a causal effect of skin penetration. This trial can be considered as an efficacy trial although most acupuncturists would consider the intervention and the whole setting as less than 'ideal'. Keep in mind that the definition of efficacy refers mainly to drug trials where highly standardized conditions make it indeed more likely to

Table 2.2 Comparison of a typical explanatory efficacy trial and a typical pragmatic effectiveness trial (based on Zwarenstein et al. 2009)

	Explanatory efficacy trial minimizing bias and maximizing internal validity but usually with low external validity (Linde M et al. Cephalalgia 2005)	Pragmatic effectiveness trial with high external validity but fewer precautions against bias (Vickers A et al. 2004)
Question	To investigate whether normal (skin penetrating) acupuncture is more efficacious in reducing menstrually related migraine than sham acupuncture without skin penetration	To investigate whether a policy of "use acupuncture" in patients with chronic headache was more effective (and cost-effective) than a policy of "avoid acupuncture."
Setting	One specialist migraine clinic in Gothenburg, Sweden	12 separate sites consisting of a single acupuncture practice and two to five local general practices in the UK
Participants	28 women with menstrually related migraine. Multiple other inclusion and exclusion criteria	401 adult patients with chronic headache. Wider inclusion and exclusion criteria
Intervention	Standardized point selection, stimulation, number, duration and frequency of sessions	Up to 12 individualized acupuncture treatment in a three-month-period
Control	Non-penetrating sham intervention at the same acupuncture points	Care as usual and 'avoid acupuncture'
Outcomes	Patients had to keep a detailed headache diary, 6 months follow-up	Simple diary at selected time points, quality of life outcomes, economic evaluation, 12 months follow-up
Relevance	Provides evidence whether skin penetration makes a difference	Provides evidence whether acupuncture may be an effective (and cost-effective) addition to the National Health Service

detect a difference between the drug and a placebo. For CAM treatments the term efficacy trial is often associated with a high degree of standardization, placebo or sham controls and an attempt to maximise internal validity. 'Pure' scientists like such trials because they can provide a clean answer to a clean question.

But does this help the practitioner or the politician who has to make decisions in the rather untidy real world? The trial by Vickers et al. (2004) investigated the question what difference it could make for the British National Health Service to allow interested patients with chronic headache to be given acupuncture. Multiple centres included a heterogeneous group of patients, acupuncturists were free to choose individualized treatments, and patients in the control group simply received usual care. Outcomes included simple headache-related measures but also quality of life and costs. Obviously, providers and patients knew their group allocation, and they were free to access other treatments. The results of the trial showed that acupuncture was associated with a small but probably clinically relevant benefit at a small additional cost to the health care system, but the set up of the trial leaves the results open to reporting biases and distortions due to use of co-interventions. Its internal validity is thus lower compared to that of Linde et al. Nevertheless, the sample size was large, the patient sample and the interventions reflected true practice, the follow-up period was longer – thus, it has high external validity. To the decision-maker it provides more valuable information but the 'pure' scientist may find the results questionable because the conditions were not truly controlled.

The two trials presented here are rather clear examples – many trials in the literature are difficult to classify even though a lot of CAM studies tend to belong to the group of explanatory efficacy research. Without internal validity a study is clearly worthless, but high internal validity does not necessarily mean that external validity is good. In ➤ figure 2.8 we try to summarize the main characteristics of studies with a focus on internal and external validity, respectively. Below we will briefly discuss three aspects which are crucial to external validity: selection of study participants, interventions and outcome measures.

2.3.2 Selection of study participants

> The results of a clinical trial should ideally be generalizable for all patients with a specific condition. Therefore, at best the study participants should be a representative random sample from the total population of interest.

While placebo-controlled randomized trials focussing on efficacy often have high internal validity, their participants are rarely representative. For example, many chronic conditions are particularly prevalent in older patients. However, these patients are very often excluded from such trials, mainly because comorbidities and co-interventions make a "clean" assessment difficult. In case of extremely narrow inclusion and exclusion criteria the results of a study only apply to the individuals selected.

The patient sample that is most appropriate depends very much on the question the study is addressing. If you want to investigate whether it makes sense to add acupuncture to the toolkit of interdisciplinary pain units you should get a representative sample from such units, but this study will have little relevance for family physicians. If you focus on patients actively choosing a specific type of CAM treatment your study sample should come from this group of patients but the results might again not apply to GP care.

Preferences and expectations are an important issue in CAM and it may well be that they are strongly associated with the outcomes. Therefore, trying to perform studies whose results are widely generalizable is often problematic. It is obviously much easier to get the consent of patients to participate in a study if they receive the treatment they prefer than if they cannot choose, as is the case in a randomized placebo-controlled trial. When compared to randomized trials, well-performed non-randomized trials tend to include patients more likely to represent those actually seeking the relevant treatment options in practice. Such studies tend to have lower internal but higher external validity than randomized and blinded trials.

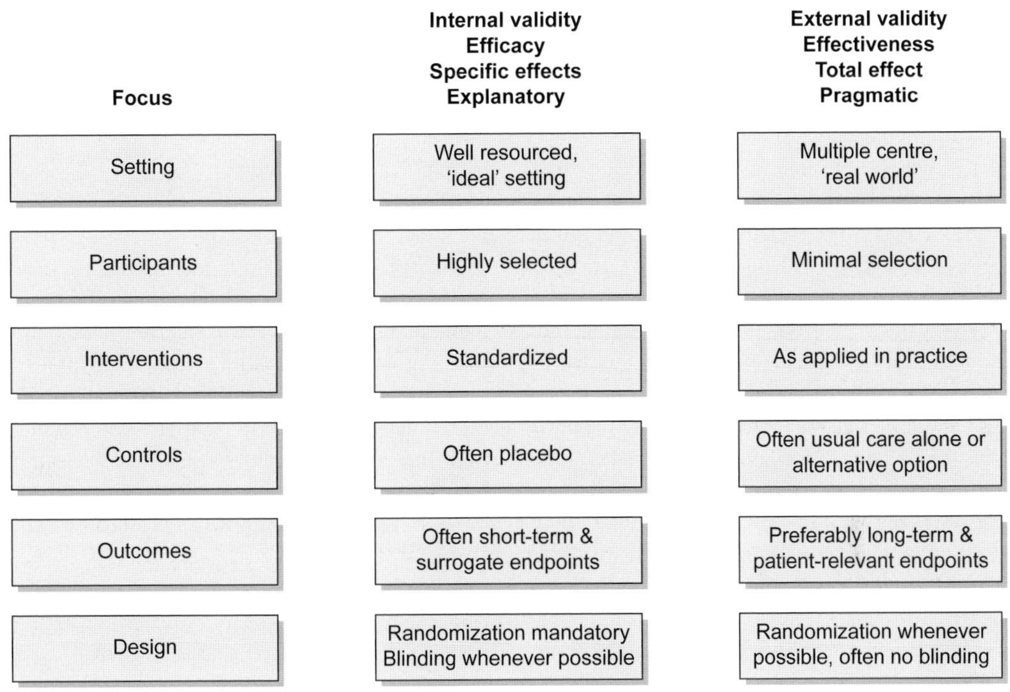

Fig. 2.8 Comparison of the characteristics of trials focussing on internal and external validity

2.3.3 Selection of study interventions

As described in chapter 1, CAM therapies are in general widely used and diversified *before* they are evaluated scientifically. Some of them are **whole medical systems** (e.g. Chinese medicine, homeopathy) that are built upon complete systems of theory and practice. As for clinical studies investigating such systems as a whole, it is difficult to provide pure scientific answers for which component has which effect, since often only a 'section' of a whole medical system is addressed in trials (for example, acupuncture out of traditional Chinese medicine). Furthermore, a number of CAM therapies have their own diagnostic classifications for customizing the individual treatment for each patient, while clinical studies usually follow a Western diagnostic approach (one treatment strategy for one Western diagnosis).

Paradoxically, in academic discussions there is a trend to generalize interpretations of CAM research findings. For example, a trial of the homeopathic remedy Arnica C30 in runners may be interpreted as evidence for or against homeopathy. Nobody would interpret a positive trial of sildenafil in erectile dysfunction as evidence for pharmacotherapy as a whole. Given the limited resources, only a tiny fraction of CAM treatments can be evaluated rigorously. Therefore, it is important to select study interventions carefully.

If a study is aiming to provide high external validity, the treatment interventions should represent what happens in routine practice.

In order to decide whether a treatment should be offered free of charge within a health system, it makes sense to perform a large multicentre trial involving a variety of practitioners and letting them do what they normally do. It is impossible to derive from such a trial whether needling in a standardized manner at defined points is more effective in reducing the frequency of migraine attacks than applying a non-penetrating sham device at the same points. However, if you do not find a difference in such a trial, does that mean that acupuncture is ineffective for headache?

It is very difficult to give general advice on how the selection of a treatment intervention for a clinical study should be made. It depends on the exact question you want to answer. There can be no doubt that in the past there have been many CAM trials in which treatments were applied in an inappropriate manner, most often to increase feasibility or reproducibility, and to facilitate the implementation of sham or placebo controls. Whatever your design, you should be conscious of the fact that you do not investigate "acupuncture" or "chiropractic" as a whole but just the intervention which is applied. Checking textbooks or establishing an expert consensus are two approaches for choosing a study intervention both for an efficacy trial with high internal validity and for an effectiveness trial with high external validity (➢ Ch. 3.3).

2.3.4 Selection of outcome measures

If you perform a trial on chronic low back pain and find that cortisol levels in blood increase by day 14 it may be an interesting and useful observation. Laboratory measures are 'objective' and not susceptible to bias and regulatory agencies often ask for evidence based on 'objective' outcomes. However, the clinical relevance of such a finding is extremely low unless it is the missing link in the evidence puzzle. In this back pain study you would normally want to know whether pain, function, need for medication and quality of life improve. And even if you find improvements after one month this is of little help if the benefits do not last for a longer period. To keep attrition low, to make measurements more objective, to decrease variability and for a variety of other reasons aimed at increasing internal validity, investigators often measure short-term effects on outcomes of questionable clinical relevance (so-called surrogate measures). If researchers decide instead to focus on long-term outcomes which truly matter, setting up a valid study often becomes difficult. For example, in research on migraine prophylaxis there is considerable pressure from the leaders in this research field to use headache diaries. Diaries are clearly the best tool to quantify headache symptoms. However, if patients have to fill in diaries over long periods of time many drop out from the study sooner rather than later because of the workload. Most trials of prophylactic drug treatments for migraine have observation periods of less than six months and still suffer from substantial drop-out rates. Long-term trials are almost non-existent. However, is it the most important issue for a migraine patient whether a drug has short-term effects (measured against placebo)? If a researcher observes patients for 24 months there will be a big problem with drop-out rates when diary entries are requested. If the researcher uses instead a simple telephone interview asking about migraine days in the last 3 months, high response rates may be achieved but the research will be criticized by the community for using an outcome measurement which is not the accepted standard.

Effectiveness trials performed to inform decision-making should investigate endpoints which are really relevant to patients. This often means that patients have to be followed up for a long time. Efficacy trials often focus on short-term endpoints which can be measured reliably but which may only be surrogates of what is really important to patients.

2.4 What study design for what purpose?

2.4.1 Studies without a control group

The study design that is most appropriate fundamentally depends on your exact research question. How such questions should be asked will be discussed in detail in ➢ Ch. 4.1. Of course, resources and feasibility also play a major role in making the choice. All the above should make clear that studies without a control group can hardly ever be used to prove the efficacy or effectiveness of a treatment. Still, we think that a study without a control group *can* be of considerable value in the evaluation of a treatment if the correct question is asked, if the study is performed rigorously and if it is reported appropriately.

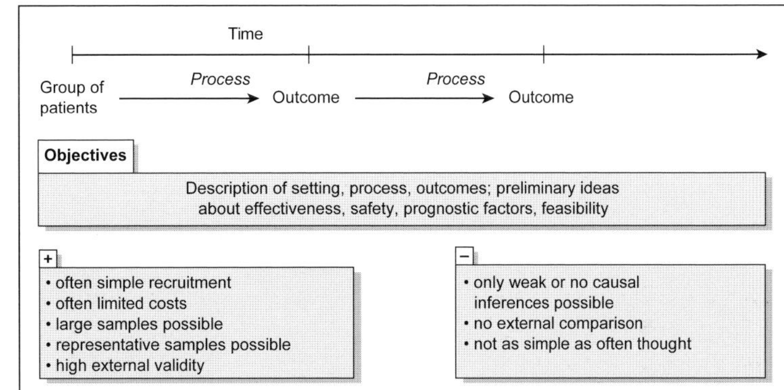

Fig. 2.9 Principle, objectives, advantages and drawbacks of prospective observational studies without a control group

Retrospective case series

When a CAM treatment has never previously been evaluated, uncontrolled studies are likely to be an appropriate first step. The most basic approach is a **retrospective case series**. 'Retrospective' means that data collected in the past are analysed. Retrospective case series only make sense if detailed and comparable information for all included cases is available. For example, a practitioner may use a standard routine in following up his patients with breast cancer with careful documentation of histological diagnoses, standard therapy and CAM interventions applied, regular follow-up visits with blood sampling and questions about side effects and fatigue. Based on this data it is possible to get an idea whether something dramatic and unexpected may have happened; or one might get an idea whether there is something worthy of further investigation. Very often, however, the routine documentation available is insufficient to draw any conclusions. Diagnostic data are incomplete, co-interventions are not documented, follow-up is short and assessments of health status are insufficient.

Prospective observational study (without control group)

Therefore, whenever possible you should do a study prospectively.

The most important type of clinical studies without a control group are prospective observational studies. Prospective means that you first define your aims and methods, and then you include, treat and observe your patients (➤ Fig. 2.9). Observational means that you do not interfere or interfere only minimally with routine practice (e.g. by setting minimal standards in the diagnostic process).

If a prospective observational study without a control group claims that its main aim was to evaluate the effectiveness of a treatment, it is very probably a bad study, or at least misleading in its report. Examples of this are many post-marketing studies (also called phase IV studies) sponsored and performed by pharmaceutical companies. In these studies physicians often include and treat a large number of patients, do some very basic documentation, and receive a sizeable fee. The main reason for performing such studies is to get providers familiar with a product. This abuse is a shame because the method clearly has some important potential. Below we give some examples on how such studies can provide useful information.

Prospective observational studies for describing settings, processes, and outcomes, and for formulating preliminary ideas about effectiveness (generating hypotheses)

Prospective observational studies can often recruit relatively easily a large number of patients who receive the target intervention in routine care, and can be performed with limited resources. Large multicenter observational studies with wide inclusion criteria offer a great possibility to gather information on how and for whom a treatment is provided, whether it is well tolerated, what the outcomes are and, possibly, whether it *may* be effective and whether it should be evaluated in further controlled studies. One such example is a large German study which involved over one hundred homeopathic physicians who included almost 4,000 consecutive new patients undergoing a first detailed homeopathic case-taking (Witt et al. 2005). Progress over several years was documented for all patients meeting very basic inclusion criteria and regardless of the conditions, treatment and outcomes. Particular emphasis was given to achieving high follow-up rates. This study provided detailed information for the first time on who seeks classical homeopathic care in Germany, how frequently patients see their homeopath, and which remedies are prescribed in what dosage (potencies). Both after the treatment and at long-term follow-up the majority of patients reported clinically relevant improvements. This does not prove effectiveness! But given that most patients had long-standing symptoms it seems reasonable to assume that the homeopathic treatment process may have been beneficial to some extent. This study provided reliable information on patients, treatment processes, the course of patient-reported outcomes – and some hints that homeopathy may be effective and that it may be worth doing studies with control groups. Drawbacks in this study are that the natural course of symptoms (in spite of the chronicity of most patients' problems), regression to the mean (in spite of some analyses trying to adjust for that), the possible use of effective co-interventions and biased reporting cannot be ruled out. And obviously it is impossible to say what element of the therapy may have been responsible for the improvements.

Sometimes prospective observational studies with a focus on observing 'treatment effects' are called **prospective case series** or **outcome studies**. There are no clear definitions for these terms. The term prospective case series is often used for smaller, less formal studies. The term outcome study was originally used to designate studies (both controlled and uncontrolled) which aimed at measuring outcomes relevant to patients, but has been used in CAM research for some time now for pragmatic, larger observational studies (sometimes with a non-randomized comparison group). Another term for prospective observational studies (with and without a control group) is **cohort studies**. The term refers to the fact that a group of individuals (a cohort) is included and observed over a period of time. However, the term is mainly used in epidemiology for studies addressing etiology and prognosis (➢ Ch. 12) and less commonly for studies evaluating treatment interventions.

Investigating safety

The most important data on safety comes from case reports and simple, large prospective observational studies. How can that be? In principle, safety is a causal question, and therefore randomized trials should be the best tool for its evaluation. In fact, the question whether a treatment is generally well tolerated can be well investigated in randomized trials. The proportion of patients terminating treatment or dropping out because of side effects is a simple and straightforward indicator. However, severe adverse effects usually occur too infrequently to be observed and detected as causally related to the interventions in randomized controlled trials. For example, while acupuncture is clearly associated with some minor unwanted effects that occur rather frequently (e.g needling pain, temporary deterioration of symptoms or autonomic reactions), severe events such as pneumothorax, infection or cardiac tamponade are of greater concern but occur rarely. The occurrence of such events has been shown in simple case reports. The causal link was – at least for most cases of pneumothorax and cardiac tamponade – so obvious that there can be no doubt that acupuncture *can* be dangerous. Prospective observational studies have, however, shown that these events occur very rarely. In Germany the rate among physicians was less than 1 pneumothorax in 100,000 patients and no cardiac tamponade in more than one million patients (Weidenhammer et al. 2007, Witt et al. 2009).

Interactions between St. John's Wort extracts and other drugs are another good example why randomized trials often do not provide relevant safety information. St John's Wort extracts have been tested against placebo or synthetic drugs in more than 50 trials, mostly for depression but also for some other related mental problems. In these trials patients with severe co-morbidities are almost always excluded and there is a careful control of concomitant medication. In the 1990s several case reports and case series became available showing that the use of

St. John's Wort extracts was associated with a drop in the plasma levels of cyclosporine and other immunosuppressant drugs given to patients with kidney transplants to prevent organ rejection. Further research proved that many St. John's Wort extracts induce the metabolism of many drugs in the liver.

The systematic monitoring of a pharmaceutical drug, device or therapy after it has been released on the market is called **surveillance** or **postmarketing surveillance**. Surveillance is typically planned prospectively. But while 'normal' observational studies include individuals meeting defined inclusion criteria, regardless of the outcomes, surveillance is more of a monitoring system which aims to make sure that relevant cases of adverse effects are not missed.

Investigating prognostic factors

Large prospective observational studies are also a good method for investigating the association between prognostic factors and clinical outcomes. For example, Weidenhammer et al. (2006) performed a large multicenter observational study of patients receiving acupuncture for chronic pain from primary care physicians. The primary aim of the study was to describe patients, processes and outcomes, but in exploratory analyses the authors examined whether outcomes differed between physicians with short and long training, between physicians with different specializations or between female and male physicians.

Preliminary studies

The term **pilot study** is used if a study is explicitly used as preparation for a more definitive study. Pilot studies can be uncontrolled or controlled, and they can be observational, experimental (the study investigates a 'model', i.e. the conditions of the study differ significantly from routine practice) or in a grey area in between. Pilot studies are used to get an idea whether a study is feasible and whether outcome instruments measure what they are supposed to measure, and may provide a rough idea of what effects might be expected.

Quality improvement

Audits are a tool for investigating whether a change in practical organisation or clinical practice makes a difference. In such a study one typically observes the feature of interest for a given period of time (e.g. outcomes in a group of patients or practice management for the reduction of waiting times). Based on these observations the process of interest is assessed and changes are introduced (e.g., adding a new therapy or changing the organisation of the practice). After a fixed time the observation is repeated to check whether the desired improvements occurred. One could argue that this study has an intrinsic control group but we prefer to keep it in this section.

2

2.4.2 Studies with a non-randomized comparison group

Why do studies with non-randomized comparison group?

Even in situations where control or comparisons groups are available, randomization is not always possible or appropriate.

For example, randomization is occasionally very difficult because of strong preferences. Anthroposophic medicine is a complex system of theories and treatments based on a specific philosophy. While anthroposophic physicians use a lot of conventional therapies, in addition they use special therapies (eurythmic movement exercises, art therapy, rhythmical massage therapy) and special medications. For "non-followers", many aspects of anthroposophy appear strange. The personal decision to rely primarily on anthroposophic medicine is a very deliberate one. If a study aims to compare the effectiveness of a complex anthroposophic approach to a standard drug treatment in patients with depression a randomized trial will be practically impossible. Most followers of anthroposophic medicine as well as those who do not follow this practice are most likely to refuse consent to randomization as the respective "opposite" treatment option does not fit their individual preference.

Randomization is not *appropriate* for the comparison of anthroposophical and conventional care if we are primarily interested in differences regarding preferences, experiences, processes and compliance, and if comparative effectiveness is only a secondary objective. Randomization is usually also not *necessary* to find out whether treatment effects are very different – if the study is well-done in other respects. If one intervention performs much worse (or much better) than the other it can usually be seen in well-executed non-randomized studies.

Wellperformed non-randomized comparative studies can have high external validity because they closely reflect usual practice. Recruitment is normally easier than for randomized trials because patients can choose their preferred treatment option. This commonly makes non-randomized studies easier to perform.

However, if allocation is not randomized it is almost inevitable that the patients in the intervention and control groups will be different. As described in ➢ Ch. 2.1.2, differences in outcomes between the groups may then be due to confounding factors. Thus the internal validity is low, or at least less certain, than in a randomized trial.

Even though frequently discussed, non-randomised comparisons are not very common in CAM research. This is probably due to three factors: 1) it is difficult to design non-randomized trials, analyze and interpret really well; 2) there is a strong emphasis on high internal validity when studies on the effectiveness of CAM treatments are discussed in the scientific community; 3) funding agencies and the industry usually prefer randomized trials.

Historical or concurrent comparison

Comparison groups for non-randomized studies can be historical or concurrent. Historical means that that the data have been collected in the past. Concurrent means that the data are collected prospectively and in parallel with the intervention group.

Historical control groups can be collected from the literature. However, this means that only data already compiled are available and that these data were collected in a different time period. It is preferable to have individual patient data instead of aggregated data from earlier studies. In recent years a large number of registries have been established, particularly in oncology but also for a number of other relevant conditions, for the surveillance of adverse effects, or in a very broad way by some insurance companies. Some of these registries contain high quality data. However, their usefulness for evaluating the effectiveness of CAM treatment is limited as the focus is usually on major conventional treatments (such as surgery, radio- or chemotherapy) and hard major outcomes (survival, major events etc.). Registries can also be used for concurrent controls if the data is collected in parallel with the study of interest. More typically in CAM research, non-randomized studies are prospective studies with parallel groups.

Matching or adjustment of confounders

As stated above, baseline differences are almost inevitable in non-randomized studies. The two main methods to cope with this problem are matching and statistical adjustments.

> Matching means that before you start the analysis you form pairs or groups of patients who are identical or as similar as possible regarding relevant factors and you exclude patients for whom matching is not possible.

In analyses with statistical adjustments mathematical procedures are used to correct (adjust) for differences in patient characteristics and baseline values.

Matching can be used in retrospective analyses of existing data, in prospective studies or in situations where you collect data for one group of patients prospectively and take data for the other group from an existing database. For example, Grossarth-Maticek and Ziegler (2007) searched a database of women suffering from cervical cancer for patients who had received treatment with mistletoe and those who had not. They then formed pairs of patients who had the same tumor stage and grading at first diagnosis, similar time since diagnosis, similar age at diagnosis, and similar conventional treatment. After forming these pairs they compared survival times between the two groups. In another study Gerhard et al. (1993) prescribed individualized homeopathy to 21 women who were diagnosed with unexplained infertility or sterility and followed them up for an extended period. From a database with 600 women treated conventionally at the same institution they selected 21 women matching for age, duration of childlessness, type of sterility, uterine, tubal, andrological factor, body mass index and type of menstrual disorder.

Matching has immediate appeal to the clinician: it sounds simple and straightforward. Instead of trusting in randomization or in analyses with complex statistical adjustments, one can directly ensure that patients are similar for some important aspects. It can be used even when the populations from which the pairs are drawn are very heterogeneous. However, matching has severe drawbacks. Firstly, it is inefficient. In most cases the data from the majority of patients cannot be used because matching patients cannot be identified. To make matching feasible the number of matching factors must be very limited; otherwise only few pairs will be identified. Secondly, the prognostic factors which really predict the outcome need to be known.

Therefore, matching as the sole strategy for creating comparable groups should be used only in exceptional cases, e.g. if statistical analyses adjusting for baseline differences and confounders are not possible and the circumstances make matching a good option (for example, availability of large databases).

The great advantage of using multivariate statistics to adjust for baseline differences or confounders is that all available data can be used. Therefore, we strongly recommend using this approach instead of matching wherever possible.

For example, a parallel study on homeopathy aimed to investigate the effectiveness, safety and costs of homoeopathic versus conventional treatment in usual care in a prospective multicentre comparative observational nonrandomized study (Witt et al. 2009). 135 children (homoeopathy n = 48 vs. conventional n = 87) with mild to moderate atopic eczema were included. The primary outcome was a validated dermatitis score at 6 months. Further outcomes at 6 and 12 months also included quality of life of parents and children, use of conventional medicine, treatment safety and disease-related costs. All children recruited into the study were included in the analyses. At baseline children in the two groups differed significantly regarding the dermatitis score and a number of other variables. To take these potential confounders into account the authors used complex statistical models and calculated adjusted differences between the groups.

This study is a good example of the possibilities, strengths and limitations of non-randomized comparisons. Homeopathy and conventional treatments were investigated in their natural environment although the inclusion criteria were relatively narrow. Part of the outcome assessment was performed by a blinded assessor, the follow-up was long, co-interventions and costs were documented carefully. The analysis was performed with up-to-date statistical methods. Even so, the observed differences regarding outcomes remain difficult to interpret due to pertinent differences in characteristics and baseline values between the groups.

In some cases it may be advisable to combine matching and multivariate statistics with adjustments. This is often done in classical epidemiology case-control studies (➤ Ch. 11). Test cases and controls are matched according to a few crucial variables to make the study feasible. Other potential confounding factors are then taken into account in the statistical analysis.

The principle, objectives, advantages and drawbacks of prospective non-randomized studies with a concurrent comparison with adjustment for confounding are summarized in ➤ figure 2.10.

2.4.3 Randomized trials

What are randomized trials?

The randomized controlled trial (RCT) is clearly the most reliable tool when it comes to the question whether the difference in the outcomes of two or more study groups is due to the treatment. Usually groups are similar at baseline, and the assessment of causality and statistics are, in principle, straightforward. However RCTs are always *experiments* because the process of randomization makes them fundamentally different from routine practice. This is also expressed by the word trial; the term randomized study is rarely used. The term 'controlled' is less clear. Does it mean that these trials have a control group, or more generally that conditions are con-

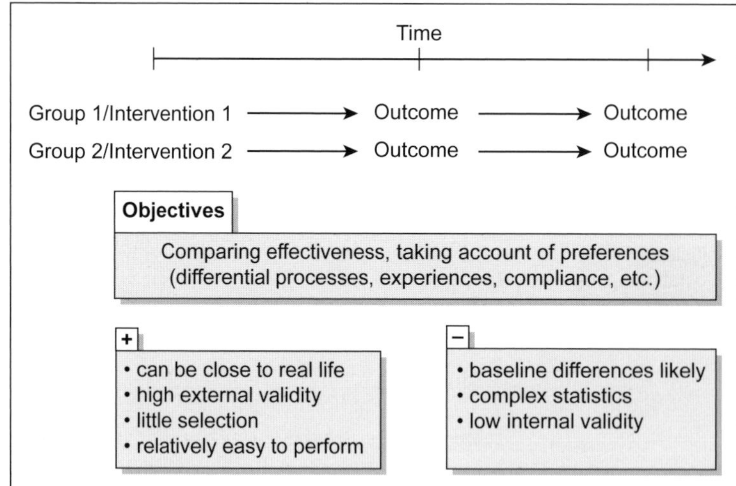

Fig. 2.10 Principle, objectives, advantages and drawbacks of prospective studies with a non-randomized comparison group (with adjustment for confounding)

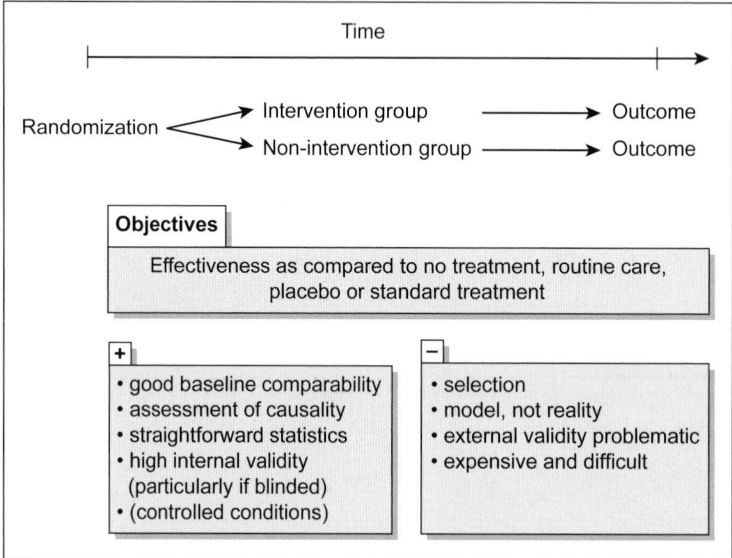

Fig. 2.11 Principle, objectives, advantages and drawbacks of randomized controlled trials (RCTs)

trolled, that is, not only variables are kept identical in all the groups but they are also standardized as much as possible? The first would be trivial; the second would fit well for explanatory trials, but less for pragmatic trials. This is why the latter are often called pragmatic clinical trials and the word controlled is left out.

From what we have written so far in this chapter it should be clear that there are many different types of RCTs: efficacy and effectiveness trials; explanatory and pragmatic trials; trials evaluating total effects (vs. no treatment, usual care alone), specific effects (vs. placebo or sham) or comparative effectiveness (vs. another therapy); blinded and unblinded (open or open-label) trials. Efficacy trials are often explanatory, blinded and placebo-controlled while effectiveness trials are often pragmatic, open and address total effects or comparative effectiveness. But there are no fixed boundaries and real trials often mix different aspects.

Randomized trials – especially efficacy trials – are often logistically complex and cost a lot of money, partly because they demand more stringent regulations for quality assurance than other studies (➢ Fig. 2.11).

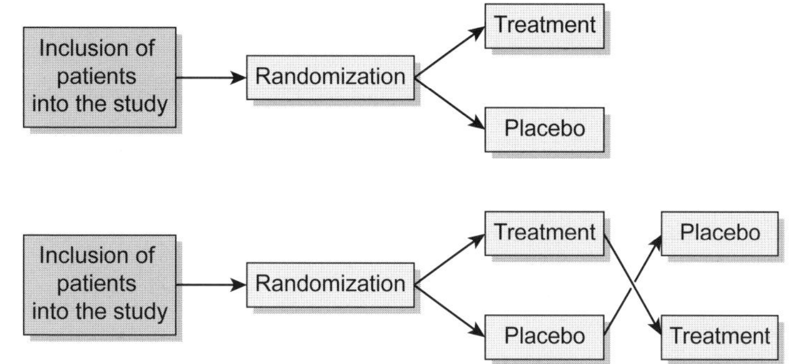

Fig. 2.12 Parallel (upper part) and cross-over (lower part) RCTs

2

Parallel and cross-over trials

RCTs can be performed as parallel or cross-over trials. Most common are parallel trials in which each individual is randomized to receive either treatment A (e.g., the intervention) or treatment B (e.g., placebo). In a cross-over trial each individual receives both treatments but the sequence of treatments is randomized (➢ Fig. 2.12).

Cross-over trials have two related advantages: they need a smaller number of patients and each patient is his/her own control. However, cross-over trials are possible only if after stopping a treatment the outcome measure returns to the baseline level. If a treatment has lasting effects or if a condition is improving or deteriorating spontaneously, the use of a cross-over design is inappropriate. If a treatment has effects which last only for a limited period of time it is possible to include a **wash-out phase** during which participants do not get any treatment.

Two-armed trials and trials with more than two arms

The most commonly used type of RCT is a two-armed (= two groups) parallel trial, but there are also many trials with more than two arms (➢ Fig. 2.13).

For example, one could perform a trial to investigate both the specific and non-specific effects of a treatment by including both a placebo and a no treatment control group (A in ➢ Fig. 2.13). You check first whether your treatment is better than doing nothing and then whether it is also superior to placebo (you may also check whether there is a relevant placebo effect). Such trials are quite commonly performed in acupuncture research as it is suspected that many sham interventions have both some physiological effects and strong psychological effects.

In drug research you quite often find trials in which a new drug is both compared to a drug already used for the condition and placebo (B in ➢ Fig. 2.13). Typical examples are a number of trials in which St. John's Wort extracts are compared both to a standard antidepressant and a placebo. At the same time, such trials investigate whether the St John's Wort extract as well as the standard antidepressant are superior to placebo and whether there are relevant differences between St. John's Wort and the standard antidepressant. This is a strong design. If there is no relevant difference between the two treatments and both are not superior to placebo you have to conclude that the trial lacks **assay sensitivity** or that the standard antidepressant is also not effective. Without a placebo group you would have concluded that both treatments are similarly effective.

If you are interested in the effects of two or more treatments or influencing factors and the combination of treatments, **factorial designs** are used. The simplest form is the 2 × 2 factorial design (C in ➢ Fig. 2.13). For example, Valerian and St. John's Wort are sometimes used in combination for some patients with depression. You could do a trial where one quarter of the patients receive both Valerian and St. John's Wort, one quarter Valerian and placebo, one quarter St. John's Wort and placebo and one quarter only placebo.

These are only examples. There are many variations. Trials with more than two arms allow the in-

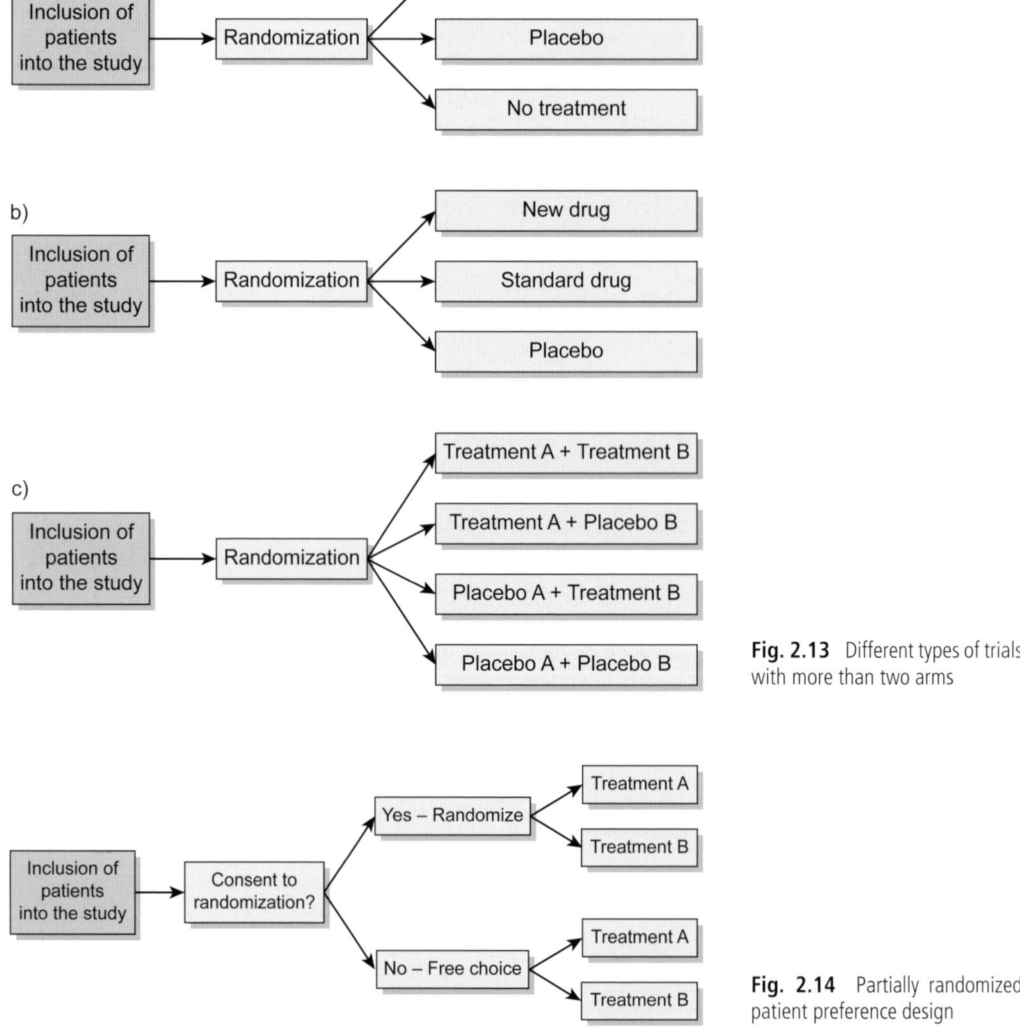

Fig. 2.13 Different types of trials with more than two arms

Fig. 2.14 Partially randomized patient preference design

vestigation of more than one answer at a time and this makes them very interesting. However, they are more difficult to design, perform and analyse than two-armed trials.

Randomization and preference

Although it is desirable to randomize for the sake of internal validity, in order to make sure that groups in a controlled study are as similar as possible, it can cause problems for external validity. If preferences have a significant influence on whether patients participate in a trial and whether they respond to treatment, the findings of RCTs may not apply to those patients who actively seek alternative options in practice. Several designs have been developed to investigate whether preferences matter. The most important is probably the **partially randomized patient preferences design** (➤ Fig. 2.14).

In such a study you ask the patients included in the study whether they have a preference for one of the two (or more) treatments or whether they agree to be randomized. Those not giving consent to randomization receive the treatment of their choice, those without preference are randomized. In this way you can check whether the results observed among your randomized patients also apply to those with a preference. If such a study includes all patients eligible for one of the two treatments it is called a **comprehensive cohort study design**.

A number of large trials have been performed in Germany on acupuncture using a variation of this design including incentives to motivate patients to accept randomization. Patients who were interested in receiving acupuncture for chronic pain conditions could choose: if they agreed to be randomized to either receive acupuncture immediately or in three months, they did not have to make the usual payment for treatment. Those who declined randomization and preferred to pay got acupuncture immediately (Witt el al. 2006). A number of other creative possibilities is possible.

So far, surprisingly, the available evidence does not indicate a strong influence of preferences. However, many trials investigating preferences had a small sample size and the analysis of such trials is much more difficult than that of usual randomized trials.

2.5 Establishing an evidence picture

We hope that this chapter has shown that a number of different designs and design variations are available. The choice of the most appropriate and feasible approach will depend on the research question asked (➤ Table 2.3). Every design has strengths and limitations. Randomized trials are the best tool to investigate whether a treatment is effective, but there are a number of additional approaches if randomized trials are not feasible. Studies without a control group and studies with a non-randomized comparison group are particularly valuable to describe what is happening in routine practice. Studies with a non-randomized comparison group can also be used, with some limitations, for assessing aspects of effectiveness. Whenever possible, it is desirable to have evidence emerging from several types of studies – hopefully producing a consistent evidence picture.

Table 2.3 What design for which question? – Summary

	UC	nrC	RCT
How is it used?	XX		
What for ist it used?	XX		
Why is it used?	XX	X	
By whom?	XX	X	
Is it safe?	XXX	X	X
Is it effective?	(X)	X	XXX
Is it value for money?	(X)	X	XXX
Has it specific effects?			XXX
How does it work?			(X)

UC = studies without control group,
nrC = studies with a non-randomized comparison group,
RCT = randomized controlled trial

REFERENCES

Benedetti F. Placebo effects. Understanding the mechanisms in health and disease. Oxford: Oxford University Press, 2008.

Conway PH, Clancy C. Comparative-effectiveness research – implications of the Federal Coordinating Council's Report. N Engl J Med 2009;361:328–330.

Di Blasi Z, Harkness E, Ernst E, Georgiou A, Kleijnen J. Influence of context effects on health outcomes: a systematic review. Lancet 2001;357:757–762.

Fønnebø V, Grimsgaard S, Walach H, Ritenbaugh C, Norheim AJ, MacPherson H, et al. Researching complementary and alternative treatments – the gatekeepers are not at home. BMC Med Res Methodol 2007;7:7.

Gerhard I, Reimers G, Kellr C, Schmück M. Weibliche Fertilitätsstörungen – Homöopathie versus Hormontherapie. Therapiewoche 1993;43:2,582–8.

Grossarth-Maticek R, Ziegler R. Prospective controlled cohort studies on long-term therapy of breast cancer patients with a mistletoe preparation (Iscador). Forsch Komplementmed. 2006;13:285–92.

Last J, Spasoff, RA, Harris S. A Dictionary of Epidemiology. Oxford, Oxford University Press, 2001.

Linde M, Fjell A, Carlsson J, Dahlöf C. Role of the needling per se in acupuncture as prophylaxis for menstrually related migraine: a randomized placebo-controlled study. Cephalalgia 2005;25:41–47.

MacPherson H. Pragmatic clinical trials. Complement Ther Med 2004;12:136–140.

2

McGauran N, Wieseler B, Kreis J, Schüler YB, Kölsch H, Kaiser T. Reporting bias in medical research – a narrative review. Trials 2010;11:37.

Moerman DE, Jonas WB. Deconstructing the placebo effect and finding the meaning response. Ann Intern Med 2002;136:471–476.

National Center for Complementary and Alternative Medicine: What is CAM? nccam.nih.gov/health/whatiscam/overview.htm. 2009.

Schwartz D, Lellouch J. Explanatory and pragmatic attitudes in therapeutical trials. J Chronic Dis 1967;20:637–648.

Shapiro AK, Morris LA. The placebo effect in medical and psychological therapies. In: Garfield SL, Bergin AE, eds. Handbook of psychotherapy and behavior change. New York: Wiley;1978:369–410.

Vickers AJ, Rees RW, Zollman CE, McCarney R, Smith CM, Ellis N, et al. Acupuncture for chronic headache in primary care: large, pragmatic, randomised trial. BMJ 2004;328:744–747.

Walach H, Falkenberg T, Fønnebø V, Lewith G, Jonas WB. Circular instead of hierarchical: methodological principles for the evaluation of complex interventions. BMC Med Res Methodol 2006;6:29.

Weber UJ, Lüdtke R, Friese KH, Moeller H. Naturheilkundliche versus konventionelle Therapie der akuten Sinusitis. Eine Pilotstudie. In: Albrecht H, Frühwald M (eds). Jahrbuch Karl und Veronica Carstens-Stiftung, Band 6, 1999. Essen: KVC Verlag, 2000, 137–151.

Weidenhammer W, Menz G, Streng A, Linde K, Melchart D. Akupunktur bei chronischen Schmerzpatienten. Behandlungsergebnisse-Rolle des Akupunkteurs. Schmerz 2006;20:418–432.

Weidenhammer W, Streng A, Linde K, Hoppe A, Melchart D. Acupuncture for chronic pain within the research program of 10 German Health Insurance Funds – Basic results from an observational study. Complement Ther Med 2007;15:238–246.

Witt CM, Brinkhaus B, Pach D, Reinhold T, Wruck K, Roll S, Jäckel T, Staab D, Wegscheider K, Willich SN. Homoeopathic versus conventional therapy for atopic eczema in children: medical and economic results. Dermatology 2009;219:329–340.

Witt CM, Jena S, Selim D, Brinkhaus B, Reinhold T, Wruck K, Liecker B, Linde K, Wegscheider K, Willich SN. Pragmatic randomized trial evaluating the clinical and economic effectiveness of acupuncture for chronic low back pain. Am J Epidemiol 2006;164:487–96.

Witt CM, Lüdtke R, Baur R, Willich SN. Homeopathic medical practice: long-term results of a cohort study with 3,981 patients. BMC Public Health 2005;5:115.

Witt CM, Pach D, Brinkhaus B, Wruck K, Tag B, Mank S, Willich SN. Safety of acupuncture: results of a prospective observational study with 229,230 patients and introduction of a medical information and consent form. Forsch Komplementmed 2009;16:91–97.

Zwarenstein M, Treweek S, Gagnier JJ, Altman DG, Tunis S, Haynes B, et al. Improving the reporting of pragmatic trials: an extension of the CONSORT statement. BMJ 2008;337:a2390.

CHAPTER

3 Basic statistics

3.1 Why statistics?

After collecting measurements from several observations, we have to find ways of displaying and summarizing the data. Statistical methods are used for this. There are simple statistical methods, such as adding values and dividing them by the number of subjects to derive the mean, or more complicated statistical methods such as logistic regression models.

For example, after measuring the blood pressure in 100 patients we may want to know the average (mean) blood pressure of these patients. Statistics can also help us to get an idea whether we observed a true effect or whether our results may have been influenced by an element of chance.

This chapter gives an introduction to basic statistics. We will demonstrate how to summarize and display your data. In addition we will give an overview about hypothesis testing which is used to compare different groups or values within one group

!

It is important to involve a statistician as soon as you develop the design of your study and not just after the data have been collected because errors or flaws in design, collecting or processing your data can be difficult or impossible to correct. But keep in mind that this chapter cannot substitute for a comprehensive textbook on statistics.

Nevertheless, understanding the basics of statistics will enable you to understand your results and help you to enter in discussions with your statistician. The second part of the book (➢ Ch. 6) will provide guidance through your own data analysis.

3.2 Types of variables and their distribution

The term **variable, or parameter, or measure** is used for the type of information such as age or severity of back pain that is assessed in your study. The **value or observation** is the data for this variable (e.g. 58 years of age). You can have different values for different time points (e.g. systolic blood pressure at 3 months–160 mmHg and at 6 months–142 mmHg). There are variables which consist of text (e.g. nationality) instead of values.

There are two main types of variables: categorical and continuous.

3.2.1 Categorical variables

Categorical variables are either **ordinally or nominally scaled**. Nominally scaled variables have multiple unordered values, whereas ordinally scaled variables have ordered categories with the interval size between these categories not being fixed. This means that the difference between two categories is not equal among all categories. For example, the difference between „slight improvement" and „great improvement" is not standardized. Other examples of ordinal variables are graduations on a scale (e.g. strong improvement/slight improvement/no change/slight aggravation/strong aggravation) which are often used in questionnaires or disease stages (e.g. asthma stage I–IV).

For variables on a nominal scale it is impossible to put the categories in an order (e.g. discharge as green/yellow/bloody). Simple types of categorical variables are **dichotomous** variables. They can only have two values (e.g. male/female or yes/no).

Table 3.1 Examples of variables and their scales

Variable	Category		Comment
Age (in years)	continuous		
Age groups (< 40, 40–60, > 60)	categorical	ordinal	
Gender	categorical	nominal, dichotomous	
Nationality	categorical	nominal	
Blood pressure (in mmHg)	continuous		
Blood pressure (below/above 120 mmHg)	categorical	nominal, dichotomous	
SF-36 Summary Scores (quality of life)	categorical	ordinal	analyzed as continuous
Numeric Rating Scale (Box with 0–10 numbers)	categorical	ordinal	often treated as continuous variable
Satisfaction with treatment (very high, high, moderate, low, very low)	categorical	ordinal	
Visual Analogue Scale (line from 0–100 mm)	continuous		

3.2.2 Continuous variables

Continuous variables appear on a continuous scale (e.g. blood pressure), where the size of a specific interval is the same regardless where on the scale the interval is taken from.

Compared to categorical variables, continuous variables usually provide more detailed information (e.g. systolic blood pressure = 155 mmHg). Furthermore continuous variables can be transformed easily into a categorical variable (blood pressure ≥ 120 mmHg yes/no), whereas it is not possible to turn a categorical variable into a continuous one.

3.2.3 Categorical or continuous?

Sometimes it can be difficult to differentiate clearly between categorical and continuous variables. For categorical variables you should typically calculate frequencies (the number of observations per category) or percentages. However, for some variables it is more common to calculate measures that are normally used for continuous variables (e.g. the mean). School grades and psychometric scales such as validated questionnaires are good examples (most have categorical single items but are analyzed as the sum of the scores). In many scales, the single items are assessed with ordinal variables (e.g. strong improvement – slight improvement – no change – slight aggravation – strong aggravation), however when calculating the summary score of the questionnaire each answer is replaced with a figure (e.g. 3 for no change).

This shows that there is a 'grey area' between ordinal categorical and continuous variables. From a conservative point of view, some ordinally scaled variables are categorical, however, they are often analyzed as continuous variables. When deciding about variables and how to display your results, you should keep this in mind. ➤ Table 3.1 gives you examples for variables and their category.

3.3 Summarizing your data

According to the type of data, there are different ways to summarize it.

Dichotomous variables can be summarized in **frequencies** (e.g. the number of subjects with a positive outcome) and **proportions** (e.g. the number of subjects with positive outcome divided by the number of all subjects and multiplied by 100 to give percentages).

For **nominal and ordinal variables** you can calculate frequencies and proportions for each category.

Continuous data are summarized in a different way:

- The arithmetic **mean** represents the average and is the typical value at the center of a set of values. You can calculate the mean by adding all the values together and dividing the result by the number of values.
- The **median** represents a 'middle value' and can be found by ordering the data from the smallest to the biggest. The median is then the observation at the center when the data set is arranged in order. When the number of values in the data set is odd the median will be the middle value. When the number of values in the data set is equal the median will be the mean of the two middle values.

The following example shows the difference between mean and median.

3.3.1 Calculating the mean and the median

Calculating the mean

Considering that 5 patients had the following values for pain severity on a 0–10 visual analogue scale

Patient 1	2.1
Patient 2	1.2
Patient 3	1.4
Patient 4	1.3
Patient 5	1.5

To calculate the mean you divide the sum of these values by the number of observations:

The sum is 2.1 + 1.2 + 1.4 + 1.3 + 1.5 = 7.5

The mean is the above sum divided by 5: 7.5/5 = 1.5

Calculating the median

If you want to calculate the **median** you have to order the values from the smallest to the largest: The median is the observation in the centre: **1.4**

Patient 2	1.2
Patient 4	1.3
Patient 3	**1.4**
Patient 5	1.5
Patient 1	2.1

If you had observed an additional value of 3.3, i.e. an even number of observations, the median would be the average of the two middle values **1.4** and **1.5** : **1.45**

Patient 2	1.2
Patient 4	1.3
Patient 3	**1.4**
Patient 5	**1.5**
Patient 1	2.1
Patient 6	3.3

3.3.2 The distribution of your data

The **distribution of the data** is important because it determines the method of analyzing your data. For **continuous data** the distribution can be visualized by the frequency of subjects for each range of values and is best displayed in an histogram.

- For **normally distributed** variables the histogram will show a symmetric bell shape (➢ Fig. 3.1 left)
- Any deviation from that shape would indicate **non-normally distributed** (skewed) variables, for example a skewed shape (➢ Fig. 3.1 right).

If distribution is skewed the mean and median will differ. This is depicted in the histograms below (➢ Fig. 3.2).

Therefore, if the data are not normally distributed the median is often the better description of the center of the distribution.

To draw a histogram you will have to specify the number of bars to be used (most software will suggest a default number). Sometimes it is useful to categorize values (e.g. age groups in blocks of five or ten years), so that you have meaningful value ranges and

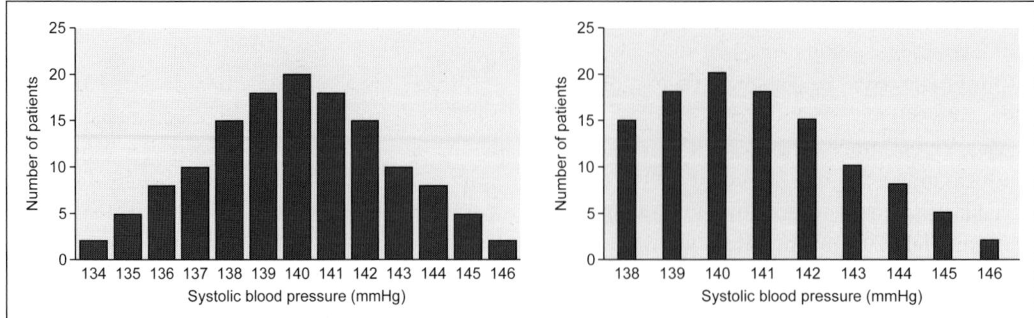

Fig. 3.1 Histograms of normally distributed and non-normally distributed data

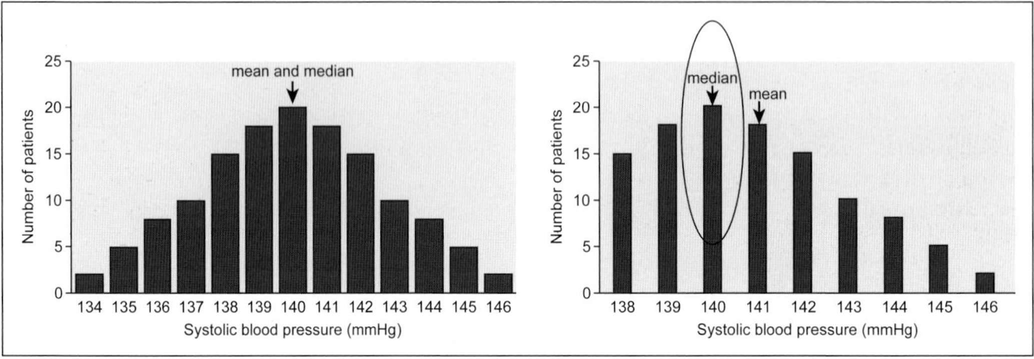

Fig. 3.2 Histograms with mean and median in data sets that are normally and non-normally distributed

a useful number of bars. If your values are spread over a large range (e.g. for age) and you have only a small number of patients for each year a clear shape of the curve might not be apparent. If too few bars are used; the shape of the curve may be lost. There is no fixed best number of bars to be used; usually 10 to 20 bars are suitable (also depending on the range of your values and the number of patients).

3.3.3 Measuring variation within your study population

A measure of **variability** for a set of data values is a number that conveys the idea of the spread for the data set. The **range** is given by the difference between the largest and the smallest values of the data set and does not use any further information. But the range not useful in all circumstances as it is strongly influenced by outliers; there is an alternative.

Recall that the **median** was a measure which splits the ordered values of a variable in half. Splitting these variable values into four quarters will yield the **quartiles**:

- The **lower quartile** (or 25 % quartile or 25th percentile or Q_1) is the cut off for the lowest quarter of the data,
- while the **upper quartile** (or 75 % quartile or 75th percentile or Q_3) is the cut off for the highest quarter of the data. The median can also be called the 50 %-quartile.
- The difference between the 75 % and the 25 % quartile is called the **interquartile range** (IQR) and is a measure of variability. Unlike the range, it is not influenced by outliers.

Variance and **standard deviation** are two further parameters for the spread of values, providing information about how the data vary around the **mean**. Most commonly used is the **standard deviation**, which is simply the square root of the variance:

- If all observations have the same value, the standard deviation will be zero, i.e. no variability at all.
- A small standard deviation indicates that the values are clustered closely around the mean.
- A large standard deviation indicates that the values are spread far from the mean

Variables that are normally distributed will have approximately 70 % of the values within plus/minus one standard deviation from the mean, and 95 % within plus/minus two times the standard deviation from the mean. The standard deviation is affected by outliers and is not a valid indicator for the spread if the distribution of your data is very skewed (➤ Table 3.2).

Table 3.2 Overview of measures of variation within your study population

Measure	Formula	Explanation
Interquartile range (IQR)	$IQR = Q_3 - Q_1$	The distance between the 75th percentile (Q_3) and the 25th percentile (Q_1). It is the range of the middle 50 % of the data and is not affected by outliers or extreme values.
Variance (σ^2)	$\sigma^2 = \frac{1}{n}\sum(x_i - \bar{x})^2$	A measure of the average squared distance between each data point (x_i) and the mean value ($\bar{x}$); calculated as the sum ($\sum$) of the squares of the deviations from the mean value ($\bar{x}$) divided by the sample size (N).
Standard deviation (σ)	$\sigma = \sqrt{\sigma^2}$	The square root of the variance (σ). An advantage of the standard deviation is, that it is expressed in the same units as the original observations (and the mean).

3.3.4 Measuring sampling variation

Statistical analysis summarizes data and uses the **study sample** to draw conclusions about the population from which it was collected. For example, a 'sample' might represent the back pain patients included in your study whereas the 'population' represents all patients of the population of a specific area (e.g. United Kingdom) suffering from back pain. The mean of your sample is unlikely to exactly match the mean of the entire population. A different sample would usually give a different mean. This is a consequence of the **sampling variation**, i.e. the variation between different samples from the same population. This will affect how **representative** your results will be. If you were to collect many independent samples of the same size from the same population you could calculate a frequency distribution of the means. The expected mean value of this frequency distribution would be the true population mean.

The standard deviation from the mean in these different samples is called the **standard error of the mean (SEM) or just standard error (SE)**. This is a measure of reliability and describes the precision of the sample mean in your study for the population under disease.

A large standard error indicates that your mean might be imprecise, whereas a small standard error indicates that your mean is more precise. The size of your standard error depends on the sample size of your study and the variability in the population. Therefore, the standard error of the mean is smaller if the sample size is larger and the data are less variable.

The standard error of the mean is also used in constructing a **confidence interval**. Confidence intervals (CI) for the mean define a range of values within which the true population mean is likely to lie.

3

Table 3.3 Standard error and confidence interval

Measure	Formula	Explanation
Standard error of the mean (SEM) or standard error (SE)	$SEM = \frac{\sigma}{\sqrt{n}}$	The standard error (SE) measures the precision with which a mean is estimated. It is calculated by dividing the **standard deviation** (σ) by the square root of **n** (the number of subjects in the sample).
Confidence interval for the mean (CI)	$\bar{x} \pm t_{1-\alpha/2}\frac{\sigma}{\sqrt{n}}$ (overall) $\bar{x} \pm 1.96\frac{\sigma}{\sqrt{n}}$ (95 % CI)	The confidence interval for the mean defines the range of values within which the population mean is likely to lie. ($\bar{x}$ = the mean value, t =, σ = standard deviation, n = number of subjects). Usually 95 % confidence intervals are used, where $t_{1-\alpha/2}$ is 1.96.

We can create CIs with a specified confidence (usually 95 %) by multiplying the standard error with the factor 1.96. Generally, the confidence interval extends to either side of the mean by some multiple of the standard error and is presented as two values, the confidence limits, in brackets separated by a comma. If you were to repeat a study many times, the 95 % confidence intervals would contain the true population mean on 95 % of the occasions. The following table shows how to calculate the standard error and confidence intervals for a mean (➢ Table 3.3).

3.3.5 Standard deviation, standard error and confidence interval

Standard deviation, standard error and confidence interval are distinct measures with different meanings. Standard deviation is shows variation within your study sample, whereas standard error and confidence interval show the precision of your study. Standard deviations are larger than standard errors. 95 % confidence intervals have nearly two times the size of a standard error. This is shown in the following figure (➢ Fig. 3.3).

3.4 Comparing two groups or two time points for one variable

Two different types of comparisons are common:
- values for different time points within one group (pre-post comparison)
- values from two or more different groups at the same time point (comparison between groups).

3.4.1 Calculating summary measures for dichotomous variables

For **dichotomous variables,** the relationship between the results from two groups could be presented by using one or more of the following **summary measures**:
- Absolute Risk Reduction (ARR)
- Relative Risk (RR)
- Relative Risk Reduction (RRR)
- Odds Ratio (OR)
- Number Needed to Treat (NNT)

➢ Table 3.4 shows an example while ➢ Table 3.5 explains how to calculate these statistical measures. The Number Needed to Treat (NNT) is usually calculated with respect to two interventions (e.g. treatment versus control) and is easy to understand and a helpful tool to explain study results to both medical professionals and patients.

As for the mean, confidence intervals can be calculated for each of these summary measures, and the measure should always be presented with its confidence interval.

Table 3.4 Example

	No effect	Improved	Sum
Treatment	40	60	100
Placebo (control)	60	40	100
	100	100	200
	No effect	**Improved**	**Sum**
Treatment	A	B	A+B
Placebo (control)	C	D	C+D
	A+C	B+D	A+B+C+D

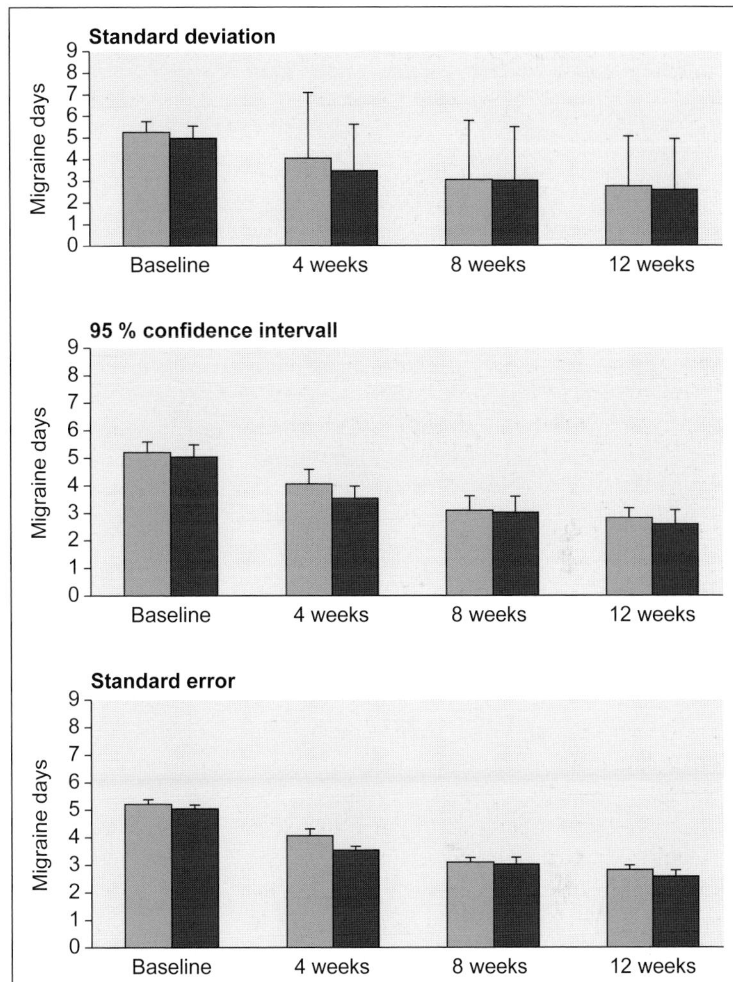

Fig. 3.3 Numbers of migraine days per month at four time points: means of two groups (acupuncture and sham acupuncture, black and white bars) with standard deviation (top), confidence interval (middle) and standard error (bottom) from the same data set (Linde K et al. 2005)

3.4.2 Calculating summary measures for continuous variables

For **continuous variables,** the relationship between the results from two groups could be presented by displaying the means of both groups or the mean difference between groups. In addition you can calculate dichotomous measures such as responder rates (e.g. patients who had 50 % improvement from baseline to 3 months on the pain VAS are counted as responders) and use the summary measures for dichotomous variables.

3.4.3 Testing a hypothesis

Hypothesis testing is an important part of study planning and analysis. It involves different steps throughout your whole study.

!

The selection of hypothesis depends upon the study objectives. In clinical research, commonly considered hypotheses include point hypotheses testing for equality, which will be described here and is often referred to as hypothesis testing for statistical superiority, and interval hypotheses testing for equivalence/non-inferiority (➤ Ch. 3.9).

Table 3.5 Statistical measures for dichotomous variables

Measure	Formula	Explanation
RR	(A/A+B)/(C/C+D)	**Relative risk** is the ratio of the 'risk' of benefit/event due to the treatment. A RR of 1 means there is no difference in risk between the two groups. A RR of < 1 means the event is less likely to occur in the treatment group than in the control group. A RR of > 1 means the event is more likely to occur in the experimental group than in the control group.
OR	(A/C)/(B/D)	Describing the strength of association or non-independence between two binary variables. Used as an estimate of the RR. The **Odds Ratio** is defined as the ratio of the odds of a benefit/event occurring in one group to the odds of it occurring in another group.
ARR	C/C+D – A/A+B	The **Absolute Risk Reduction** is the percentage by which your therapy reduces the risk of a negative outcome.
RRR	(C/C+D) – A/ A+A)/C/C+D or ARR/(C/C+D) or simple 1 – RR	The **Relative Risk Reduction** is calculated by dividing the absolute risk reduction by the response rate (% of patients with positive treatment response) of the control group. The relative risk reduction can be more useful than the absolute risk reduction in determining an appropriate treatment plan, because it accounts not only for the effectiveness of a proposed treatment, but also for the relative likelihood of an incident (positive or negative) occurring in the absence of treatment.
NNT	The NNT is the inverse of the ARR: NNT = 1/ARR = 1/(C/C+D – A/A+B)	The **Number Needed to Treat** is the number of patients you need to treat to prevent one additional undesirable outcome (death, stroke, etc.). If a drug has an NNT of 50, this means 50 people need to be treated with the drug to prevent one additional undesirable outcome compared to the control group. NNT are always rounded up to the nearest whole number.

When planning your study you must define your hypothesis. When planning the statistical analysis it is important that you (or better, your statistician) choose the right statistical test. You have to ensure that during your study the necessary data are collected from your study population. Then you can calculate the value from the specific test statistic for your null hypothesis and the p-value. Finally the p-value is compared to the pre-specified significance level (usually 5%) and the results must be interpreted.

You can use hypothesis tests to determine for example whether means or proportions differ significantly between groups (e.g. an acupuncture group and an exercise group after 3 months of treatment) or within one group but at different time points (e.g. after 3 and 6 months of acupuncture treatment). A statistical hypothesis always consists of a **null hypothesis** (H_0) which usually assumes no effect (e.g. there is no difference between the two treatment groups for the severity of back pain) and an **alternative hypothesis** (H_A) which holds the null hypothesis not to be true (e.g. there is a difference between the two treatment groups for the severity of back pain).

- H_0 for back pain after 3 months: mean pain score in acupuncture group = mean pain score in exercise group
- H_A for back pain after 3 months: mean pain score in acupuncture group ≠ mean pain score in exercise group

The alternative hypothesis usually contains the situation that you want to prove. You will then test the null hypothesis and if a **significant difference** is found you can reject the null hypothesis.

Since you can never be 100% certain that the results will only be in one direction (e.g. the pain intensity in group A will definitely be lower than in group B) you should usually use a **two-sided-test** (or two-tailed-test). If you decide to use a **one-sided-test** (or one-tailed-test) you should use half of the significance level of 5% that is typically used (i.e. use 2.5%).

!

In reality, one-sided-tests are rarely used. Even if you have a strong expectation that your study treatment will not be worse than the control intervention, you cannot be completely sure that this is correct and that your data will show it.

3.4.4 Relevance of the p-value

The primary aim of **hypothesis testing** is to provide a **p-value** which helps you to make a decision about your hypothesis. In statistical hypothesis testing, the p-value is the probability of obtaining your data (or more extreme data), given that the null hypothesis is true. You use the p-value to accept or reject your null hypothesis.

!

The smaller the p-value, the greater is the evidence against the null hypothesis.

You must decide before performing a test how much evidence you require to reject the null hypothesis. In medicine, the usual convention is to consider that a p-value below 0.05 gives sufficient evidence to reject the null hypothesis. In this case the results are said to be 'significant at the 5% level'. This leaves only a 5% chance that you made a mistake in rejecting your null hypothesis. In some cases you may require stronger evidence and use a cut-off point of $p < 0.01$.

If the p-value is 0.05 or above, the usual conclusion is that there is insufficient evidence to reject the null hypothesis. In this case your results would be considered not significant (at the 5% level). This could mean that with a p-value of 0.04 you would reject the null hypothesis whereas with a p-value of 0.06 you would not have enough evidence to reject the null hypothesis.

However, failing to reject the null hypothesis does not necessarily mean that the null hypothesis is true; there might simply be not enough evidence to reject it, for example because your sample size is too small. The terms **'significant'** and **'highly significant'** are often seen in papers but are not usually defined in statistical textbooks. It is important to remember that the choice of a significance level of 5% is arbitrary, yet needs to be specified in advance.

!

To present your results only with a certain cut-off, i.e. simply stating in a manuscript that 'p = ns' or '$p < 0.05$' can be misleading. To be transparent you should therefore always quote the original p-value from your statistical test (e.g. $p = 0.048$ instead of $p < 0.05$).

Sometimes a p-value near (but above) the significance level (e.g. $p = 0.068$) is interpreted as a trend. However, most medical journals are very conservative and interpret a p-value above 0.05 as not significant.

!

Please note: hypothesis testing is used in confirmatory testing of one predefined primary endpoint; however, statistical tests are often also used in a more exploratory way.

Returning to the p-value, another important aspect is that the p-value does not relate to the **clinical importance** of a finding. For example, since the p-value depends to a large extent on the sample size of the study, a large study might find a small but clinically unimportant difference which is significant with a very small p-value, whereas a small study might find a large difference that is clinically important but not statistically significant. Clinical importance describes that the difference between for example two treatments or two time points has a relevant size. The effect should be noticeable for the patient. For example a study on low back pain has shown that acupuncture reduces the pain intensity by 5 mm more than physiotherapy. The scale used was a 100mm Visual Analogue Scale and patients stated at baseline an average pain intensity of 56 mm. Five mm on this scale is a small difference and most patients might not even recognize it. Whereas 20 mm which represents more than 30% pain reduction compared to baseline would be a more relevant effect.

The p value is based on test statistics and the choice of the most appropriate **statistical test** for the results of your study depends on

- the type of variable (outcome and explanatory variables)
- the distribution of your data
- whether your outcome is dependent or independent

- the number of groups in your study.

You already know that you could have **continuous** or **categorical variables** and a categorical variable could be dichotomous, nominal or ordinal (➤ Ch. 3.2).

3.4.5 Statistical tests for comparing means

From your descriptive analysis you have the information for each continuous variable as to whether the data are approximately **normally distributed** or not:

- If the data are normally distributed, you can use so called parametric tests (such as t-tests)
- If not normally distributed, you should use non-parametric tests.

Another important aspect is whether your data are **dependent (paired)** or **independent (unpaired)**. Imagine a study with observations of the same patient at multiple time points (e.g. 3 months, 6 months and 12 months):

- Repeated observations of the same patient are **dependent**, because the same patient is more likely to respond in the same way to an intervention than a different patient is. If you do not take into account the correlation of repeated observations, your results will be inaccurate. Because of this, you have to use statistical tests that take this correlation into account.
- Observations from different patients are usually classified as independent.

➤ Table 3.6 gives an overview of appropriate statistical tests for a comparison of observations from two independent or two dependent, groups.

Table 3.6 Statistical tests for comparing means

Outcome variable	Independent observations	Dependent observations
Ordinal variable (e.g. age groups)	Mann-Whitney test (= Wilcoxon rank-sum test)	Wilcoxon signed rank test
Continuous variable (e.g. blood pressure in mmHg)		
• Normally distributed	Unpaired t-test	Paired t-test
• **Not** normally distributed	Wilcoxon rank-sum test	Wilcoxon signed rank test

3.4.6 Statistical tests for comparing proportions

The aim of some studies is to compare two proportions, for example the proportion of responders under two different treatments, or the proportion of patients who experience a certain event (e.g. stroke) in two groups. To test whether two proportions differ significantly, the chi-square test can be used. It can also be employed when you have more than 2 groups.

However, the chi-square test for 2 groups requires a sample size that should be at least 20, approximately. If you have smaller data sets, Fisher's exact test is more appropriate. For dependent data McNemar's test and Bowker's test of symmetry are available (➤ Table 3.7).

Table 3.7 Statistical tests for comparing proportions of categorical variables

Outcome variable	Independent observations	Dependent observations
Dichotomous variable (e.g. gender)	Chi-squared test or Fisher's exact test	McNemar's test
Dichotomous variable for small sample size	Fisher's exact test	(exact) McNemar's test
Nominal with more than 2 values (e.g. ethnicity)	Chi-square test	Bowker's test of symmetry

3.4.7 Confidence intervals

Confidence intervals are also helpful for interpreting your data and making a decision. In contrast to hypothesis tests, confidence intervals do not provide a p-value. However, they quantify the result of interest (e.g. the difference of means) and help you to assess the clinical implication of your study results. The relationship between the confidence intervals for the difference of two means and the statistical test is that if a 95 % confidence interval does include zero (for means) or one (for ratios), the p-value will be >0.05 (i.e. not significant).

The standard practice should be to report both confidence intervals and a p-value, in order to provide the magnitude and precision of the effect.

3.4.8 Type I and type II errors

There could be **errors in the decision when you do hypothesis testing** despite your best efforts to conduct a sound study. You need to take two possible errors into account:

- **type I error** (or alpha error)
- **type II error** (or beta error).

The type I error gives you the likelihood of rejecting a "correct" null hypothesis and the type II error the possibility of not rejecting a "false" null hypothesis.

The maximum possibility of making a type I error is denoted by your significance level of alpha (usually 5 %). Remember to predefine the significance level when planning your study.

The possibility of making a type II error is denoted by beta, while its complement (1-beta) is called the **power** of the test. The power of a test is the probability of rejecting the null hypothesis when it is false. In other words, the power gives, as a percentage, the likelihood of detecting an existing treatment effect. Thus your power should be as high as possible; however, there is always a small chance of making a type II error (➤ Ch. 4.9).

!

The power of a study is important: To have a 'good' chance to detect a real treatment effect, the power of your test should be at least 70–80 % but preferably 90 % or 95 %.
Undertaking a trial with a lower power could be ethically irresponsible because involving patients in a study which has a priori not enough power to detect the effect might put patients at risk without any benefits.

There are some **factors that influence the power of a test**. The power increases with:

- larger sample size
- smaller variability of the observations
- larger significance level
- larger effects.

3.4.9 How to deal with multiple testing

Usually your study includes a number of different outcomes and you want to make several comparisons using statistical tests. Although all tests formally aim to test a hypothesis, it is important to **differentiate between testing your main hypothesis** (usually you have one or two hypotheses) and **additional tests which are helpful for interpretation** (most of the tests).

For example, using statistical tests to detect significant differences in further endpoints could be helpful (e.g. your primary endpoint was back pain measured on a VAS, but you also evaluated back function and quality of life). However, these tests are **exploratory** and should only be used for orientation, whereas your predefined primary test is **confirmatory** and can be used to confirm your results.

If you would like to test more than one hypothesis on a confirmatory level it can result in **multiple hypothesis testing**. The problem of multiple testing is that the type I error rate increases, in proportion to the number of comparisons. If you use a significance level of 5 % and perform one test you can be 95 % sure that you don't reject the null hypothesis wrongly. If you perform 20 tests because you have 10 endpoints and measured them at 3 and 6 months, at least one of your p values will be false positive with a probability of over 60 %.

You have three main options for solving the problem of multiple testing:

- **defining a single primary endpoint,**
- **using a hierarchical test procedure,**
- **adjusting for multiple testing.**

The most common method is to define one **primary endpoint** (primary comparison) *a priori* when planning your study.

However, if you have a study where two endpoints are similarly relevant (e.g. symptoms and use of medication in patients with allergic rhinitis), or where you compare three groups (e.g. Hypericum, placebo and conventional antidepressants) you have to consider the other options.

For a **hierarchical test procedure,** you must rank the planned tests in a suitable order a priori, and then only perform each test on your chosen significance level (usually 5 %) as long as the previous test was significant.

For example, in a 3-arm trial your first step is to test for the primary outcome 'pain severity after 2 months' between acupuncture and waiting list group (H_0: there is no difference in pain severity after 2 months between acupuncture and waiting list group). If there is a significant difference you are allowed to perform the next test for a second null hypothesis (H_0: there is no difference in pain severity after 2 months between acupuncture and sham-acupuncture group). If there is no significant difference you have to stop the confirmatory testing. Further tests could only be done on an exploratory level.

3

If you decide to **adjust for multiple testing** then among the easiest and most commonly used approaches are Bonferroni and Bonferroni-Holm procedures.

Bonferroni multiplies each p-value by the number of tests carried out and the interpretation of the results is based on these adjusted p-values. For example, if you had two primary endpoints (back pain and back function) and the p values are 0.015 and 0.034, after adjusting the p values according to the Bonferroni approach they will be 0.030 and 0.068. Using a significance level of 5% there would still be a significant difference for back pain but not for back function. Bonferroni is an easy but rather conservative approach.

Bonferroni-Holm is a more commonly used method. It performs simultaneously more than one hypothesis test by placing the p values into an order. For example: four null hypothesis are tested with $\alpha = 0.05$. The four unadjusted p-values are 0.01, 0.03, 0.04, and 0.005. The smallest p value is 0.005. Since this is less than 0.05/4, null hypothesis four is rejected (which means its alternative hypothesis can be accepted). The next smallest p-value is 0.01, which is smaller than 0.05/3. So, null hypothesis one is also rejected. The next smallest p-value is 0.03. This is not smaller than 0.05/2, so in this case you do not see evidence to reject the null hypothesis at the level of $\alpha = 0.05$. As soon as that happens, you stop the procedure. Therefore, for the hypothetical hypotheses one and four in this example you were able to detect a significant difference on a confirmatory level ($\alpha = 0.05$), while for hypotheses two and three this is not the case.

!

Keep in mind that you usually perform a number of statistical tests: for your secondary endpoints, for your baseline characteristics, for several time points and maybe for more than two groups. They will all be presented in your paper. It is thus very important to distinguish between your primary and secondary endpoints and to describe all comparisons for the secondary endpoints as exploratory.

3.5 Comparing more than two groups for one variable

If you want to perform a statistical analysis that is more complicated, for example you want to compare more than two groups or have different time points, or want to adjust for possible confounders, you have to use a **statistical model**.

3.5.1 Statistical models and tests for comparing more than two groups for one variable

One method known as the **one-way analysis of variance (ANOVA)** is used to test for differences among two or more groups. If you are comparing only two groups the regular t-test and the ANOVA give the same results. The method is called one-way ANOVA because the groups are classified by just one variable, for example a treatment variable with 4 different values (placebo, waiting list, medication A and medication B). This procedure is adequate if the outcome data are continuous and normally distributed.

Although ANOVA is relatively robust for moderate deviations from normal distributions, if the data are quite skewed or the variance in the treatment groups differs, you must transform the data or use the non-parametric Kruskal-Wallis test. The Kruskal-Wallis test is an extension of the Wilcoxon rank sum test that is used to compare two or more groups for non-normally distributed continuous variables. If you have repeated measures on the same patients (e.g. back pain at baseline, 8 weeks and 6 months) you can use one-way ANOVA for repeated measures.

The following table gives you an overview about the appropriate statistical test for comparisons of two or more groups or multiple observations (➤ Table 3.8).

Table 3.8 Statistical test for comparisons of 2 or more groups or multiple observations

Variable	Independent observations of different patients	Dependent (repeated) observations of the same patients
Categorical variables		
Dichotomous variable	Chi-squared test	Cochrans' Q
Ordinal variable	Kruskal-Wallis test	Friedman test
Continuous variables		
Normally distributed	ANOVA	Repeated measurement ANOVA
Not normally distributed	Kruskal-Wallis test	Friedman test

3.6 Comparing two or more groups for more than one variable

In our data we have so called **independent variables (covariates)** that are available at the start of a study, for example, the baseline pain score, age, gender, or socio-economic status. And we have **dependent variables** that are created during the intervention process (e.g. pain score after 3 months). The covariate (independent variable) is a variable that is possibly predictive of the outcome studied (dependent variable). It may be of direct interest or it may be a confounding or interacting variable.

Depending on the context, an independent variable or covariate is also known as a predictor, regressor, explanatory or exposure variable. The dependent variable is also known as a response, measured, observed or outcome variable.

Multiple linear regression analysis allows you to investigate the joint effect of **covariates** on a **dependent continuous variable** which is normally distributed. You can predict their influence on the dependent variable and/or you can adjust for this influence and report an adjusted mean. An example is the mean of back pain in two treatment groups adjusted for gender, age and duration of disease.

3.6.1 Correcting for baseline differences

3

Multivariate statistics can correct (adjust) your mean values and p-values for a number of potential confounders (e.g. baseline values). You can choose to adjust for several explanatory variables. However, as a general rule of thumb, the number of variables should not be greater than 1/10 of your sample size.

If an ANOVA (see above) is extended to calculate corrected (adjusted) differences between two or more groups by adding additional covariates into the model, it is called **analysis of covariance (ANCOVA)**. ANCOVA can be used for example to address the problem of **confounding**, which is a relevant problem in studies (➤ Ch. 5). It is often present in non-randomized studies, but can also occur in randomized controlled trials when baseline variables of the groups are not balanced (e.g. one group is older than the other). A treatment is only certain to be associated with the outcome after all confounders (known and unknown) have been taken into account. The baseline value of your variable (e.g. pain at baseline) usually has an important influence on the result at the end of the study (e.g. pain after two months) (Vickers AJ, 2004).

!

The use of ANCOVA with the baseline values as covariates is strongly recommended in randomized controlled trials even if you compare only two groups and there were no obvious baseline differences between them, as it usually increases the power of your statistical test.

3.6.2 Logistic regression and statistical modelling

If we have a **dichotomous dependent** variable and a number of **explanatory variables**, statisticians use multiple **logistic regression methods**. This model belongs to the family of generalized linear models. To evaluate the influence of explanatory variables on the result of a dichotomous variable (e.g. 'improved' vs. 'not improved') logistic regression can be used. From the explanatory variables the category of the outcome into which each individual will fall can be predicted. The results for each explanatory variables (or 'risk factor') can be expressed by the odds ratio (OR).

Generating a mathematical model that describes the relationship between two or more variables as explained above is called **statistical modelling**. This can include linear regression, multiple linear regression or logistical regression methods, but there are many more methods and models. For more details about statistical models you should consult a statistics textbook (e.g. DuPont, 2002) or, better still, a statistician.

3.7 Analysis populations

After all the study data are collected you can analyze them for different (predefined) groups (or 'populations').

The **intention-to-treat population (ITT)** usually includes all patients who were included in your study with the intention that they should receive one of the study interventions including that of the waiting list group (e.g. all randomized patients). The ITT analysis is recommended because it includes also the data of drop outs or those patients who used co-interventions. This leads to smaller treatment effects, but reflects usual care.

The **per-protocol population (PP)** includes only patients who followed the study protocol sufficiently. You should decide in advance and state in your protocol the main criteria for your study participants to be included in this population. This analysis provides you with information about the effect under ideal (but maybe not realistic) conditions. In addition, the baseline balance between groups aimed for by the randomization process might not be present in the PP-population.

The **'complete cases analysis'** is another option. This refers to an analysis where only data from those ITT-patients who provided information at all measurement time points were included.

!

The analysis based on the ITT-population (ITT analysis) should be the primary analysis for all studies that seek to show a superiority of one treatment over another treatment. The PP analysis will be a secondary analysis and provides additional information. However, in studies that have a non-inferiority (or equivalent) hypothesis, an ITT analysis is not always considered the best option (explanation about non-inferiority ➤ Ch. 3.9).

3.8 Dealing with missing values

In clinical research, **missing values** are a common occurrence, because not all patients complete their questionnaires or show up for all study appointments. Missing value means that no data value is stored for the current variable.

The validity of your study results will depend (among other things) on the completeness of your data set. If not too much data are missing, then statistical methods can be helpful to estimating (imputing) these missing data. Several statistical methods have been, or are currently being, developed to deal with this problem (Donders et al., 2006; Twisk, 2002).

In general it is good practice to substitute (impute) your missing data.

One imputation method is the **last value carried forward (LVCF)** method. This means that the value from an earlier measurement time point is transferred to the following missing one. However, if a disease is progressive, such as dementia, these values might be too optimistic.

There are more conservative techniques which substitute some value for a missing data point, e.g. mean substitution. Once all missing values have been imputed, the data set can then be analyzed using standard techniques for complete data.

While many imputation techniques are available, two examples are hot-deck imputation and regression imputation:

- **Hot-deck imputation** fills in missing values on incomplete records using values from similar, but complete records of the same dataset.
- In **regression imputation,** the data from the complete records are used to estimate a regression equation of the complete data on the vari-

able with some observations missing. Then the predicted mean from this equation is substituted for each missing value.

Another technique is called **multiple imputation** which can be based on hot-deck, regression imputations or others. Here, each missing value is replaced with two or more imputed values. With this procedure, multiple imputed data sets are generated. Each one is now complete and can be analyzed. The results are then pooled to derive a mean result across all data sets. Analysis with any kind of imputation technique for missing data could be used as primary or as sensitivity analysis. This should also be defined a priori in the study protocol.

3.9 Interval hypotheses: equivalence/non-inferiority and superiority

Most randomized controlled studies follow a so-called 'point' null hypothesis. This is generally the case if you are comparing a treatment with a waiting list or a placebo intervention. Here you will test for equality and reject the null hypothesis when you find a statistically significant difference, and therefore accept the alternative hypothesis. This is usually referred to as test for statistical superiority (➢ Ch. 3.4.3). However, for some comparisons, for example a new treatment vs. a standard treatment, it is interesting to use 'interval' hypotheses. Here you can look for **non-inferiority, clinical superiority** or **equivalence** based on predefined clinically important differences. You should have some prior knowledge about your test intervention, because for non-inferiority and clinical superiority you test only in one direction, whereas for equivalence you test in both directions.

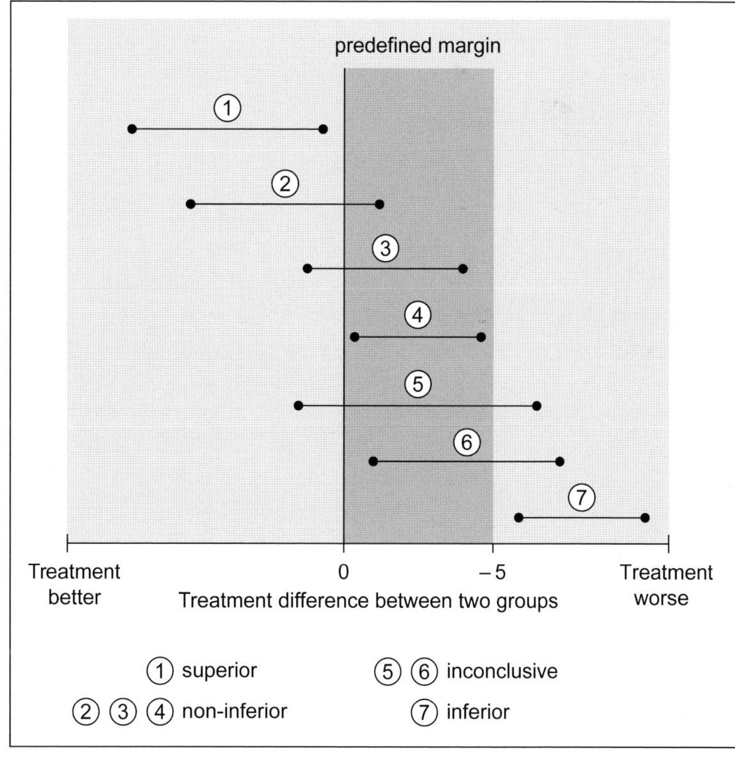

Fig. 3.4 Decision for non-inferiority, superiority, or inferiority based on confidence intervals for a difference between two treatments

3

> **!** For all interval hypotheses you have to predefine interval limits which serve as margins for a clinical important difference.

The non-inferiority hypothesis can be very useful when comparing a complementary or alternative medicine (CAM) treatment with a conventional standard treatment since the aim might be not to prove that a CAM-treatment is better, but to prove that it is not substantially less effective (but maybe more effective) than a standard therapy. Although the rationale for such trials occurs frequently, non-inferiority or equivalence trials are still rare in the medical literature. In addition, for a non-inferiority trial you have to predefine the margin for the non-inferiority, which usually represents the smallest value for a clinically relevant effect. Overall, a confidence-interval based approach is often used to interpret results from non-inferiority and equivalence trials. The interpretation of the results depends on where the confidence interval lies relative to both the margin of non-inferiority and the null effect. For two-sided evidence (equivalence trials) you have two margins (one above zero and one below) and both need to be considered. The different scenarios are shown in ➢ figure 3.4.

In superiority trials, an intention-to-treat-analysis is recommended because it leads to smaller treatment effects than per-protocol-analysis and so prevents any overestimation of the treatment effect. However, in non-inferiority or equivalence trials an intention-to-treat analysis could increase the type I error (leading to a false conclusion of non-inferiority or equivalence). A analysis based on other populations (e.g. complete cases, per protocol) might be desirable (Piaggio G et al., 2006).

> There are special statistical tests for testing the interval hypothesis. In addition special methods are required for the sample size calculation in such trials. You should discuss this with your statistician.

REFERENCES

Donders AR, van der Heijden GJ, Stijnen T, Moons KG. Review: a gentle introduction to imputation of missing values. J Clin Epidemiol 2006 Oct;59(10):1,087–91.

DuPont WD. Statistical Modeling for Biomedical Researchers: A Simple Introduction to the Analysis of Complex Data. Cambridge University Press, Cambridge 2002.

Linde K, Streng A, Jürgens S, Hoppe A, Brinkhaus B, Witt C, Wagenpfeil S, Pfaffenrath V, Hammes MG, Weidenhammer W, Willich SN, Melchart D. Acupuncture for patients with migraine: a randomized controlled trial. JAMA. 2005;293(17):2,118–25.

Piaggio G, Elbourne DR, Altman DG, Pocock SJ, Evans SJW. Reporting of noninferiority and equivalence randomized trials: An extension of the CONSORT statement. JAMA. 2006;295:1,152–1,160).

Twisk J, de VW. Attrition in longitudinal studies. How to deal with missing data. J Clin Epidemiol 2002 Apr;55(4):329–37.

Vickers AJ. Statistical reanalysis of four recent randomized trials of acupuncture for pain using analysis of covariance. Clin J Pain 2004 Sep;20(5):319–23.

Practice – Planning, managing, analyzing and publishing a clinical study

The second part of this book addresses practical issues of planning (➤ Ch. 4), managing (➤ Ch. 5), analyzing (➤ Ch. 6) and publishing (➤ Ch. 7) a clinical study. Within the chapters the content is presented in steps which are ordered chronologically following the usual flow of a clinical study. In addition three case studies serve as practical examples to illustrate those steps and to provide practical information on different study designs.

- Case study 1 is an uncontrolled observational study which evaluates the effects of a new acupuncture intervention in a pilot study.
- Case study 2 is a randomized double-blind placebo-controlled study comparing a herbal drug with a placebo
- Case study 3 is a pragmatic randomized study comparing acupuncture or yoga in addition to usual care with usual care only.

You will find the complete case studies in the appendix.

CHAPTER

4 Planning

4.1 Formulating the research question

This chapter helps you to develop an appropriate research question.

4.1.1 Why a clear research question is so crucial

A clinical study is nothing else but a systematic and formal approach to answering a specific question. Therefore, posing the research question appropriately is absolutely fundamental (> Fig. 4.1). There are many ways in which a study can fail to answer the question posed, but if the question asked is not well thought through and clearly stated, the study is fundamentally flawed from the beginning. A clear research question is the precondition for deciding which choice of design makes sense, which patients should be included, which interventions and controls should be discussed and which outcomes should be measured.

4.1.2 Practical steps

Formulating the research question	
Step 1	Define your interests
Step 2	Pose a preliminary question
Step 3	Check whether your question has already been answered
Step 4	Consider whether your aims are realistic
Step 5	Formulate your definitive question

Step 1: Define your interests

The aim of any clinical study must be to answer the question posed in the most reliable and valid manner possible. You have to be aware that the result of your study might be different from your expectations (in fact, this happens quite often in CAM research), and you have to take great care that your personal bias will not distort your research. However, it is legitimate to have personal, institutional, professional, financial or whatever interests, and to plan your study in such a manner as to maximise the chance to achieve your goal. Although it often seems as if science takes place in an ivory tower, researchers are human beings and embedded in their social networks. If you are undertaking a study you should be very clear why you want to do it. Are you an idealistic researcher searching for the truth? Do you want to prove to the skeptical world how wonderful your therapy is? Do you want to challenge your colleagues? Do you want a new product approved by relevant agencies? Are you aiming at achieving a degree? Is there a funding program from your government for your institution?

Your interests influence how you approach your study and which question you ask. For example, if you wanted to convince the skeptical outside world that your therapy is effective for a given condition it would not make sense to use a design which has low acceptability, such as a study with historical controls. Instead it might be necessary to answer the question whether your treatment has an effect over placebo. At the same time you should not embark on a study with overoptimistic assumptions when there is a high risk of producing a negative result. If you want to test a new product for licensing you have to be aware of all relevant guidelines and legal requirements. If you want to achieve your PhD in the next two years you should not start a study with a long-term-follow-up of several years. Many (probably most) studies take much longer than planned, so if you have restricted time and resources, do not go for the Nobel prize.

During the whole study you must be aware that your interests might bias what you observe, the decisions you make during the study and how you interpret the data. While it is legitimate to have interests and to design your study in a manner to achieve your aims, you should do everything possible to make sure that your results will not be influenced by your biases.

So consider writing your personal interests up on a sheet somewhere and re-checking repeatedly whether you are still on the right path when you progress through your study.

Step 2: Pose a preliminary question

Novices to research often come up with broad questions, such as "Is acupuncture effective for back pain?" However, such a question is too vague to guide the development of a study protocol clearly.

!

If your study is on the effects of a treatment you should ask your question in a PICO-format. PICO stands for **P**atients, **I**ntervention, **C**omparison and **O**utcome (Richardson et al. 1995).

The broad question "Is acupuncture effective for back pain?" can be the basis for a number of quite different PICO-questions. For example:

- Do patients receiving acupuncture recover faster from acute back pain than patients receiving massage?
- Does acupuncture relieve pain intensity in patients suffering from chronic low back pain more effectively than sham acupuncture?
- Do patients suffering from chronic neck pain who receive acupuncture in addition to routine care have less long-term disability than patients who receive routine care alone?

While such preliminary PICO questions still leave a lot of detail open (Will your acupuncture intervention be individualized or standardized? When will you measure the outcome?, etc.) they already give you sufficient guidance to proceed in the planning process and to focus your thinking.

Consulting published literature assists you in your aim to put questions into a PICO format. You should go to a high class journal (inferior journals sometimes have bad articles making it difficult for the reader to find out what was actually investigated) and simply look at the abstracts of randomized clinical trials. You should be able to formulate the PICO-question of the study after reading the objective and methods section of the abstract (if not, it is probably a bad study).

Some senior researchers might ask you what your hypothesis is. A hypothesis is a statement about a specific result expected under defined conditions. You can easily transform your PICO question into a hypothesis. For example, we could re-phrase our PICO question above into "We hypothesize that patients with chronic low back pain receiving acupuncture will have lower pain intensity than patients receiving sham acupuncture." Hypothesis testing is introduced in detail in ➤ chapter 3.

PICO is usually assumed to be designed for studies with a control group, but can also be applied to studies without a control group. For example, a study could investigate whether patients suffering from chronic low back pain and receiving acupuncture have less pain after the intervention compared with before the intervention. It is clear that such a study will provide much weaker evidence of effectiveness than a controlled study. Nevertheless your question should still be as clear as possible, and maybe this will lead you to decide that it is not wise to do an uncontrolled study.

What can you do if you have more than one question? In real life we would like to know not only whether acupuncture relieves low back pain intensity better than sham acupuncture, but also how it compares to standard care, whether it is better than no treatment, how long the effects last, whether deep needling is better than superficial needling and whether ten sessions are better than five. While some closely related questions can be answered within one single study (for example, whether there are short-term *and* long-term effects), you are strongly recommended to focus on one main question. Different questions usually demand several studies. In any case, whenever possible try to get your questions into a PICO format.

Obviously, there are studies in which a treatment is applied but which do not focus on treatment effects. For example, a study may investigate which types of treatment are applied to low back pain patients in chiropractic care. In these cases PICO cannot be applied.

Step 3: Check whether your question has already been answered

You might not be the first person in the world thinking about research on a particular topic. Once you have your preliminary question, the first thing you should do is to look whether others have already come up with the answer. For most clinical researchers this will mean that they check in PubMed for studies on their topic.

PubMed (www.ncbi.nlm.nih.gov/pubmed) is an electronic database provided by the US National Library of Medicine that includes over 18 million citations from the medical literature. PubMed covers most relevant scientific journals in clinical medicine and is a perfect resource for doing a fast and easy search on your topic free of charge. A short introduction tosearching in PubMed is provided in www.ncbi.nlm.nih.gov/pubmed. PICO questions can be used for PubMed searches very well (Schardt et al. 2007).

In many instances it will be sufficient to search PubMed to identify literature for your topic. Hopefully you find some studies in your area, but none which provides the answer you are searching for. You should read the most important articles carefully because this will be hugely important for your further planning. In some instances, however, you might have to go to other conventional electronic databases or specific CAM databases (➤ Table 4.1) or handsearch specialty journals. Sometimes, you find a lot of interesting material and you may even consider doing a systematic review before embarking on, or while developing, your own study (➤ Ch. 11). Sometimes you find very little.

Step 4: Consider whether your aims are realistic

After reading a considerable number of articles on your topic you hopefully find out that your question has not been answered yet. Otherwise you may modify it so that your study will provide additional knowledge. You have probably formed an idea of the problems the available studies had to cope with. In your brain the study starts to materialize. Think

Table 4.1 Databases for identifying relevant literature

Databases	Description
Other conventional databases	
Embase (Excerpta Medica database)	www.embase.com Contains over 19 million indexed records from more than 7,000 peer reviewed journals, covering 1947 to date, with more than 600,000 additions annually Subscription necessary (possibly freely available at universities)
Cochrane Library	www.thecochranelibrary.com Contains the most comprehensive collection of randomized clinical trials, 4,000 full-text systematic reviews and further 10,000 abstracts of systematic reviews Abstracts free, for full text subscription necessary (often freely available at universities)
Science Citation Index/Science Citation Index Expanded	www.isiwebofknowledge.com Also enables searching for articles that cite a defined article Subscription necessary (possibly freely available at universities)
CAM specific databases	
AMED (Allied and Alternative Medicine)	www.ovid.com/site/catalog/DataBase/12.jsp 200,000 citation from 600 journals partly accessible at universities
Hominform	www.hominform.soutron.com/homqbe1.asp specific for homeopathy free
Acubriefs	www.acubriefs.com/ specific for acupuncture currently under reconstruction
Natural Medicines Comprehensive Database	www.naturaldatabase.com/ specific for herbal medicine subscription necessary
Herbmed	www.herbmed.org/ specific for herbal medicine free
Mantis	www.healthindex.com/ focus on osteopathic, chiropractic and manual medical literature subscription necessary
CAM-Quest	www.cam-quest.org specific for clinical research in CAM/homeopathy (ca. 14,000 citations) free

carefully now whether you really think you can do your study, whether it is worth all the work, etc. Discuss your ideas with experienced colleagues. If you still want to go ahead with your study, it is now time for step 5.

Step 5: Formulate your definitive question

Put your main question (or hypothesis) into its final shape. Keep it in a PICO format whenever possible. Try to add some more detail to it (for example, whether you aim to use standardized or individualized acupuncture, at which time point you want to measure your main outcome). It might be that you have to adapt some detail of your question during the protocol development, but in general you have completed a crucial job. You have defined what type of answer you aim to provide.

4.1.3 Case studies

Case study 1: Uncontrolled observational study (pilot study)

Case study 1 is a descriptive, observational study without control group evaluating a treatment with retained acupuncture needles that stay in place for 7 days, an uncommon procedure but frequently used by one particular acupuncturist.

Step 1: Define your interests

Andrew is primarily working in practice and wants to check whether his own experiences can be verified. He does not want to convince sceptics and he has only limited resources for a study. In this situation an uncontrolled observational pilot study seems a realistic option.

Step 2: Pose a preliminary question

Does pain decrease in patients suffering from chronic low back pain when they receive the newly developed acupuncture technique?

Step 3: Check whether your question has already been answered

Andrew checks PubMed and possibly also a more specialized acupuncture database for any literature describing a technique similar to the one used by him. He finds a lot of literature on acupuncture for chronic low back pain which helps him to develop his protocol, but he does not find a study with a technique similar to the one developed by himself.

Step 4: Consider whether your aims are realistic

Andrew's main considerations are whether he will be able to recruit a sufficient number of patients and whether he is able to do all the necessary work alongside his daily practice.

Step 5: Formulate your definitive question

The question remains the same as in step 2.

Case study 2: Randomized double-blind placebo-controlled study

Case study 2 is an efficacy study performed within the relevant regulatory framework. The objective of this randomized controlled trial is to evaluate whether two months treatment with Devil's claw is more effective than placebo in patients with chronic low back pain.

Step 1: Define your interests

Betty would like to promote the integration of herbal medicine into the routine care of her own and other pain units. Her colleagues are open but sceptic. A double-blind, placebo-controlled, randomised trial seems the most appropriate way to proceed in this situation. Herbal medicine is governed by legal regulations in her country which require that such studies comply with the same standards as drug research (ICH-GCP guidelines, ➢ Ch. 4.2).

Step 2: Pose a preliminary question

Do patients suffering from chronic low back pain experience better pain relief with Devil's claw than with placebo?

Step 3: Check whether your question has already been answered

A literature search in Pubmed identifies only one placebo-controlled trial with a promising result. However, reviews conclude that further research is necessary.

Step 4: Consider whether your aims are realistic

Betty can collaborate with several other academic pain units which are willing to participate and able to recruit a sufficient number of eligible patients. However, she needs funding (public or from a manufacturer) to make sure that the trial can be performed in an appropriate manner.

Step 5: Formulate your definitive question

Do patients suffering from chronic low back pain who receive 1,500 mg of dried alcoholic extract of Harpagophytum procumbens (Devil's claw) daily for two months have lower pain intensity than patients receiving a placebo?

Case study 3: Pragmatic randomized study comparing three groups

Case study 3 is a comparative effectiveness study in a usual care setting. The objective of this pragmatic randomized three-armed trial is to evaluate whether additional acupuncture or yoga treatment is more effective than usual care alone in the treatment of patients with chronic low back pain, and whether one of these treatments is more effective than the other.

Step 1: Define your interests

Carol has an interest in this area. The subject is relevant to the health care system and public funding is available. It is important that her institute successfully competes for funding, Carol's project thus seems both interesting and promising.

Step 2: Pose a preliminary question

Do patients suffering from chronic low back pain who receive acupuncture or yoga in addition to usual care experience better pain relief than patients who receive usual care alone?

Step 3: Check whether your question has already been answered

A literature search in Pubmed identifies several trials comparing acupuncture with usual care alone and Yoga with usual care alone. No study investigated Viniyoga and there was no direct comparison of acupuncture and any Yoga technique.

Step 4: Consider whether your aims are realistic

The availability of funding and the cooperation of a sufficient number of centers seem to make a large trial feasible.

Step 5: Formulate your definitive question

Do patients suffering from chronic low back pain who receive either individualized acupuncture or Viniyoga for three months in addition to usual care have better back function than patients who receive usual care alone?

REFERENCES

Richardson WS, Wilson MC, Nishikawa J, Hayward RS: The well-built clinical question: a key to evidence-based decisions. ACP J Club 1995, 123:A12–3.

Schardt C, Adams MB, Owens T, Keitz S, Fontelo P. Utilization of the PICO framework to improve searching PubMed for clinical questions. BMC Med Inform Decis Mak. 2007;7 : 16.

Acknowledgement: We would like to thank Daniela Hacke (Carstens Foundation, Essen) for her help with the overview of the databases.

4

4.2 Study Protocol

4.2.1 What is a study protocol?

This chapter gives an introduction to the aim and the structure of a study protocol.

A study protocol is a document that describes the aims, design, methodology, statistical methods, and procedures of a clinical study. The protocol usually gives the background to and rational for the study being conducted. In addition to the study design the protocol also describes

- the types of patients required for the study
- the schedule for procedures and interventions
- details of the interventions (e.g. type, dosage)
- the duration of the study.

Developing the study protocol is a process that goes hand in hand with planning the study. The study protocol describes the whole study in detail before the study is started.

The existence of a study protocol allows researchers in multicenter studies to perform the study in exactly the same way, so that their data can be combined as though they were all working at the same site. It also gives the study administrators, as well as the local researchers, a common reference document for the researchers` duties and responsibilities during the study.
A good study protocol makes it much easier to write the final report or an article for publication.

In addition, the study protocol is often needed to apply for funding and to get approval from ethical committees or governmental boards, such as the Federal Drug Administration (FDA www.fda.gov) in the United States or the European Medicines Agency (EMEA, www.emea.europa.eu) in Europe.

The format and content of clinical study protocols sponsored by pharmaceutical, biotechnology or medical device companies in the United States and the European Union have been standardized: they are written to follow the Good Clinical Practice Guidance (ICH GCP www.ich.org) issued by the International Conference on Harmonisation of Technical Requirements for Registration of Pharmaceuticals for Human Use (ICH). Study protocols for other clinical studies do not necessarily follow the standard format.

If you want to perform a higher level study, you need a Steering Committee and a Data and Safety Monitoring Board:

- The **Steering Committee** is a group of key executives who are responsible for providing guidance on the overall strategic direction of the study. Its purpose is to set strategies and goals for the research effort and to ensure that problems are quickly identified and acted upon.
- The **Data and Safety Monitoring Board (DSMB)** is an impartial group that oversees clinical trials and reviews any severe adverse events as well as intermediate and end results and judges whether they are acceptable. This group determines when trials should be altered or terminated early.

4.2.2 Develop your study protocol – step by step

Writing a study protocol is a tedious process which can take several months. Doing it step by step can be very helpful. These are the most important steps:

Develop your study protocol step by step	
Step 1	Collect relevant information and get started
Step 2	Get advice from experts
Step 3	Use a check list
Step 4	Create a template
Step 5	Start with those parts which are clarified

Step 1: Collect relevant information and get started

The nature of the content of a study protocol is always the same; however, the structure and format depend on the aims, the sponsors and the board responsible for giving approval. Search the website of the relevant institutions and follow their guidelines. It can be helpful to get some examples of study protocols from your colleagues. Get information about the requested format (e.g. grant application or ICH-GCP format) for your study protocol. To develop your research idea search for studies published in the same research area. In addition, the CONSORT statements (www.consort-statement.org) which exist for different study types might be helpful. Although their main aim is to improve the reporting of clinical studies they can be of great value when planning your study.

Step 2: Get advice from experts

Writing the study protocol also includes reflection on your research idea. Discussing the study with your colleagues and friends is always helpful. When you decide on the details of your study (e.g. inclusion and exclusion criteria or statistical methods) you should screen the relevant literature and discuss relevant aspects with experts. For example if you are unsure about clinical parameters that may influence your decision on inclusion criteria, discuss them with an expert who has the relevant clinical expertise. Although we have described how to do a simple sample size calculation (➤ Ch. 4.9), you should consult a statistician.

> **!** Discuss any statistical methods with a statistician.

Step 3: Use a checklist

Checklists can be very helpful to prevent you forgetting important aspects.

The following checklist contains the relevant aspects and can be helpful when writing your study protocol.

Presentation

- Cover page: title, principal investigator and affiliation, sponsor, protocol version and date, RCT registration number if applicable
- Investigators: names and affiliations
- Main centers: names and affiliations
- Steering committee: names and affiliations
- Summary of the protocol (objective, study design, study population, intervention, outcomes)

Background and Justification

- Importance of subject area
- Review of relevant literature
- Study justification
- Relevant research questions
- How will the study results be used

Objectives

- Primary objective
- Secondary objectives

Material and methods

- Study design
- Study population: including inclusion/exclusion criteria (subject and disease characteristics), recruitment procedure, where the study will take place (or setting), advertising plan and, if applicable, recruitment materials
- Randomization and blinding (if applicable): generation of the randomization sequence and concealment, details of blinding
- Sample size calculation: total number and number in subgroups, include all assumptions as recalculation might be necessary
- Interventions: for drug/device studies: active study agents, placebo study agents, blinding/labeling/preparation of agents, storage, administration, toxicities and guidelines for adjustments) and for other types of intervention studies: active intervention description and control group, if applicable
- Outcomes: description of all outcomes with references
- Data collection: all study procedures, assessments, and subject activities
- Provide a schedule of all study assessments and subject activities, including a table or figure for the timeline
- Data management: coding, processing, software, validation and data cleaning (data management plan)
- Statistical analysis plan: analysis population, descriptive analysis, primary endpoint, null and alternative hypothesis, statistical procedure for primary endpoint and secondary endpoints

- Pilot studies or pre-testing, if applicable
- Validity (bias and other limitations)

Safety monitoring plan

- Definition of adverse events, serious adverse events
- Procedures that will be used to monitor subject safety
- Names of responsible people who will identify, document, and report adverse events
- Safety monitoring board or other ways to review the safety
- Rules for stopping the study with regard to efficacy and safety

Ethical considerations

- Informed consent
- Data storage and protection
- Ethical review committee

Project management

- Participating institutes and people (e.g. principal investigator, project coordinator, data manager, statistician, monitor)
- Responsibilities and tasks of each partner
- Quality assurance
- Data ownership
- Publication rights

Timetable

- First patient in
- Last patient in
- Last patient out
- Last questionnaire in
- Closing the database
- Clean file (check data for plausibility and validity)
- Data analysis
- Report/publication

Resources

- Financing the study
- Other resources

References

- Literature cited

Appendices

- Questionnaires
- Variable list with definitions
- Forms for patient information and informed consent
- Investigator's brochure

Step 4: Create a template

The length of the study protocol depends on the special requirement for your study (e.g. ICH-GCP or grant application), but you can expect to write at least 20–30 pages. Due to the fact that writing a study protocol is a process and many changes will happen a template is very helpful. Some institutions (e.g. clinical trial units) offer special preformatted templates for study protocols according to the requirements of ICH-GCP and you should check if your institution provides this service before you start.

Step 5: Start with those parts which are already clarified

There is no need to write the chapters of your study protocol in a special order. You could start with those chapters which are already clarified, for example the background and objective. In addition it can be helpful to start work early on with those chapters which include standardized definitions (e.g. safety: adverse events serious adverse events).

Once you have finalized your study protocol, add information that identifies the current version (e.g. the version number and the date).

!

> The final version should be signed before the start of your study (at least by the principal investigator and the statistician). If you change the study protocol after the study has started the changes must be highlighted as 'amended'.

This is done in a new version of the study protocol including a short summary of the changes. In addition the IRB/Ethics Committee has to be informed. You always need to check the formal requirements of the IRB/Ethics Committee which approved your study if you want to introduce any changes into your study protocol.

4.3 Interventions and Controls

4.3.1 Theoretical background

Controls and interventions are central aspects of your study. Both should already be defined in the study question. For example you might want to evaluate the efficacy of gingko biloba compared to placebo in patients with dementia. But, to define your intervention and control fully, much more detail is needed. Defining intervention and control is important and can be time consuming. This chapter will summarize these aspects.

Interventions

The intervention is the therapy you intend to evaluate. In CAM the intervention is often the driving force for doing a clinical study. You might be fascinated by a specific therapy and want to demonstrate to the scientific community that it really works. Thus you might already have a clear understanding of this intervention. However, in order to get your results accepted you should describe the rationale your intervention is based on and support it by references (e.g. from text books).

!

You should also think again about the aim of your study. If your study's focus is on efficacy you will probably develop a **standardized treatment protocol**, if the study focus is on effectiveness (in usual care) **a less standardized treatment protocol** may be more appropriate.

If you have no clear concept when you develop the details of your treatment regime you have two options. One is searching the literature and choosing an intervention which is widely accepted for the treatment of your study population. The other option is to use expert knowledge. You can get expert consensus by running consensus conferences or using the tool of written Delphi rounds or a combination of both. An expert consensus is always more powerful for gaining acceptance of your results, but you will need to get experts involved and you will have to moderate them in such a way that consensus on an intervention is achieved at the end of the process.

You will also have to think about **co-interventions**. Co-interventions are all interventions which are permitted and part of the study intervention. They depend on the disease, the duration of your study and on your study question.

4

Traditional diagnosis and individualization of interventions

In many traditional systems such as Chinese medicine, homeopathy, Ayurveda, Tibetan medicine or Japanese medicine (Kampo), the treatment is chosen following a traditional diagnosis and is individually tailored to each patient.

However, most randomized controlled trials are designed to compare two or more standardized treatments and usually do not reflect aspects of individualized treatment. If you plan a study in a traditional system (e.g. Chinese medicine pharmacotherapy) design options can be integrated into RCTs which include a traditional pattern diagnosis as well as individualized interventions.

For better communication with conventional doctors and inclusion of the results in systematic reviews and meta-analyses, you should use a conventional diagnosis as the main diagnosis. An additional traditional diagnosis can be used for choosing the appropriate individualized pharmacological treatment, for example, in Chinese pharmacotherapy for each trial patient.

The time point at which the traditional diagnosis is made depends on your study question. If you want to determine the efficacy of a drug, both groups should receive the same traditional diagnostic procedure before randomization (➤ Fig. 4.1). Designs

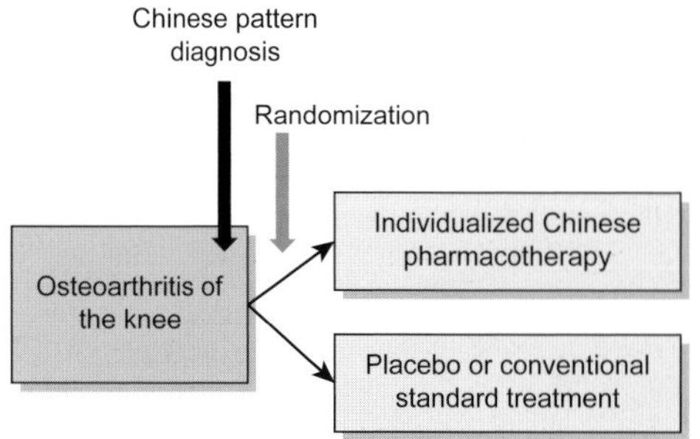

Fig. 4.1 Individualized RCT where the traditional diagnosis is separated from the study intervention

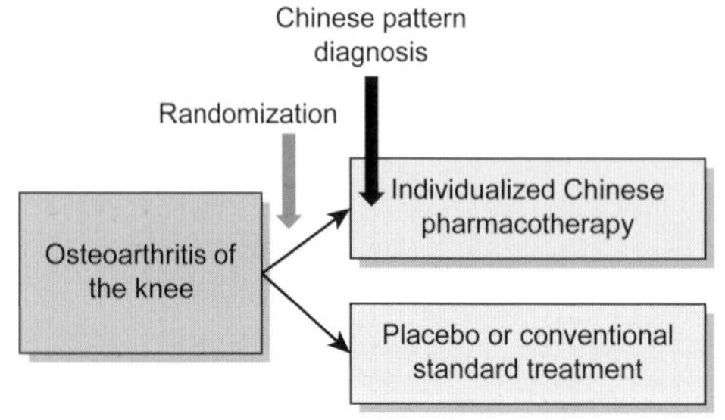

Fig. 4.2 Individualized RCT which compares Chinese medicine with placebo or conventional standard care and includes Chinese medicine pattern diagnosis in the study intervention

such as these have previously been used for homeopathy (Walach et al. 1997) and were also suggested for traditional herbal medicines (Watanabe et al., 2011).

If you want to evaluate Chinese medicine pharmacotherapy as a whole system, only those patients who were randomized to the Chinese medicine pharmacotherapy group should receive the Chinese medicine pattern diagnosis (➢ Fig. 4.2). This will ensure that both traditional diagnosis and individualized treatment will be represented in the study intervention.

After receiving individualized treatment, all patients in the traditional medicine treatment group will be analyzed as one group independent of their treatment. If you are interested in analyzing the data for each traditional diagnosis and the respective treatment separately, the traditional diagnosis can be used for stratification within the randomization process (➢ Ch. 4.4.). This trial design allows for individualized, traditional treatments according to the traditional diagnosis. However, it also means using a range of different formulae. To ensure blinding it might be necessary to prepare an appropriate placebo for each formula if they differ in appearance, smell and taste from each other. In this type of trial, the patients should not only be blinded for the treatment but they should also receive no information about their traditional diagnosis. For many Western diagnoses, more than two traditional diagnoses are common. Different patterns would result in a larger number of subgroups and some of these might be too small to have enough statistical power for a subgroup analysis. It therefore makes sense to use the pooled patterns as the primary analysis and to prespecify subgroup analysis for the more common patterns.

Another possibility, which might be easier to handle in the trial process, is to use the traditional diagnosis as an additional inclusion criterion, thus only recruiting those patients with the relevant traditional diagnosis. When using this design, you should be aware that a large number of patients may need to be screened. In addition, the results will be less representative of the Western diagnosis, and integration into conventional care might be more difficult because Western trained doctors will not be able to differentiate between the different traditional diagnoses.

Controls

The choice of the appropriate control is determined by the aim of your study and depends on your study question. You can have one or more control groups.

Study aim	**Control**
Specific effect	Placebo or sham treatment
Superiority or non-inferiority to standard treatment	Standard treatment
Effectiveness (total effect)	No treatment
As add-on that is superior to usual care	Usual care

The development of the details for the control intervention can use the same procedures as the development of the study intervention (literature search or consensus process). The following table shows examples of aims and respective control group.
Let us have a closer look for the different control group options.

Placebo control

If the aim of your study is to determine a specific effect of your intervention you must think about using a placebo or sham procedure.

The most important aspect of a placebo control is that it is **inert,** which means that it has no specific effect. This type of placebo is also called **pure placebo**. To ensure blinding and to minimize bias the placebo should be **indistinguishable** from the study intervention. Placebos are typically used in drug trials and have to be developed for each drug. Study intervention and placebo have to be indistinguishable in appearance (form, color), smell and taste. This is likely to be easy for a study on homeopathy but more difficult for a study on herbal medicine.

For herbal medicine, capsules could be an option, but keep in mind that patients might be clever and open the capsules to check for the substance. Another option is to use a very low, ineffective dose of the herbal medicine as placebo control. This would be called an **impure placebo**. An impure placebo is defined as a substance which has no effect at the used dosage for the disease studied. It could also be another herbal medicine or a conventional drug which can mimic side effects. If the study intervention has typical side effects (e.g. gastro-intestinal symptoms) this might result in unblinding.

The term **sham procedure** is used when you have a non-pharmaceutical intervention. Sham procedures mimic the study intervention, can be at least single blinded and have no specific effect. Typical sham procedures are sham operation and sham acupuncture.

Sham procedures are more complicated than placebos, because they have to mimic complex interventions such as acupuncture or massage. In most cases it is not possible to blind the practitioner, so these studies are often single-blinded. Here the example of acupuncture will be used to show the complexity. For acupuncture several sham procedures are available including both skin penetrating and non-penetrating needles (see box).

Most common types of sham acupuncture

- Standard needles inserted at inappropriate sites and/or superficially.
- Non-penetrating needles:
  1) Streitberger needle: the needle is blunt and the shaft of the needle is free to move inside the handle. When pressed on the skin, the needle appears to penetrate but the handle simply telescopes over the shaft. The needle is supported vertically on the skin by an adhesive dressing applied over an O-ring around the point,
  2) Park needle: consists of an oversize guide tube with a silicon flange which adheres to the skin by means of double-sided tape and the standard guide tube makes sliding fit within the Park tube.
- Other devices used to touch or press the skin, such as the finger-nail, an empty guide tube or a cocktail stick.

The choice of the sham-acupuncture procedure depends on your study question. Penetrating sham acupuncture aims to detect an effect which is specific for the acupuncture point tested because both the sham and the real acupuncture group penetrate the skin resulting in non-specific effects. The differences between the groups are the points used and the manipulation of the needle. In contrast, non-penetrating sham-acupuncture does not penetrate the skin and physiological effects due to skin penetration will only occur in the acupuncture group.

Although the non-penetrating sham needle does not penetrate the skin and can be used at real acupuncture points, it may still have physiological activity due to an acupressure effect. Until this is clarified, it is better to use it on sham points.

Standard treatment

A standard treatment control, often called active control, is an intervention which reflects a commonly accepted standard treatment for the disease under study, often following treatment guidelines. This control allows comparison of the study intervention with a standard treatment. In this case a non-inferiority or superiority of your study intervention is investigated as compared to the standard control. This is helpful especially for serious diseases (e.g. cancer) where placebo controls can be difficult from an ethical point of view.

However, when using standard treatments as controls, blinding can be a problem and the results of your study may thus be biased. For example if, in a back pain trial, a non-pharmaceutical treatment (e.g. Yoga) is compared with a drug (e.g. diclofenac), blinding is impossible because both interventions are easily recognized. In drug trials blinding is usually possible except when the drugs differ in size, appearance or smell. Here a **double dummy technique** can be used which is giving both a standard control and a placebo control (➢ Ch. 4.6).

4

For example, if a homeopathic treatment is compared with serotonin re-uptake inhibitors in patients with major depression, blinding can be achieved by giving all patients two types of medication (the study intervention and the placebo). For this, two different placebos have to be produced – one for the homeopathic remedy and one for the serotonin re-uptake inhibitors. Patients in the homeopathy group get the homeopathic remedy and the placebo of the serotonin re-uptake inhibitor and patients in the conventional treatment group get the serotonin re-uptake inhibitor and the placebo of the homeopathic remedy.

No treatment control

A no treatment control provides a control for the normal course of the disease. However, ethical considerations influence the feasibility of this kind of control. For example if you plan a study on patients suffering from chronic neck pain, it is unethical to leave them without any treatment for pain. A compromise is to allow some rescue medication and define it as co-intervention.

Another problem with no treatment controls is motivating the patients to be randomized if one option is just to get nothing. This can be solved by offering patients in this group the intervention at the end of the study. This is called a **waiting group control**.

!

Bear in mind that you need to have good arguments for the necessity of a no treatment control to convince Institutional Review Board (IRB)/ethics committees and to motivate patients to participate in your study.

Usual care

The term usual care or routine medical care reflects the typical care available outside a study context. If the aim of the study is to evaluate the effectiveness of an additional offer within the health insurance system, a usual care group would be the appropriate control group. However, this only makes sense if the study has a pragmatic approach and the treatment regime in the control is not standardized. Another option is to compare a standard treatment regime with usual care to assess whether a more standardized treatment regime results in a better outcome. It is important to document the care used during the study to allow a transparent description of the treatments in usual care.

4.3.2 Define your control and interventions

After deciding which type of control intervention you will use, you should define the details of your study intervention, the co-interventions allowed, and the controls. The information about intervention, control and co-intervention should be documented in the study protocol, the investigator's brochure and the patient information.

!

Keep in mind that for efficacy studies, intervention and control have to be more standardized, and for effectiveness studies less standardized.

The most important steps are:

Define your control an intervention	
Step 1	Define your study intervention
Step 2	Define your control
Step 3	Define your co-interventions

Step 1: Define your study intervention

You have already outlined the main aspects in your study question; you will now have to define the details of your study intervention. First you should choose a process to design your intervention. Your intervention should be based on literature or a clearly described consensus process. Keep in mind that you have to describe this in your publication. Whatever method you use at the end of the process you should have a clear and detailed description of your intervention. For acupuncture, herbal medicine and homeopathy the CONSORT extension for reporting results (summary in the following box) can help with the details needed for this description (for more details and examples see the original publications).

Reporting guidelines for study interventions

Acupuncture *(MacPherson H, Altman DG, Hammerschlag R, et al. Revised Standards for Reporting Interventions in Clinical Trials of Acupuncture (STRICTA): extending the CONSORT statement. Acupunct Med 2010;28(2):83–93)*

- Style of acupuncture
- Needling details (points, number of needle insertions, depths, de qi, stimulation, needle retention time, needle type)
- Treatment regime (number and frequency of treatments)
- Practitioner (training and practice experience)

Herbal medicine

Reporting Randomized, Controlled Trials of Herbal Interventions: An Elaborated CONSORT Statement. Ann Intern Med. 2006;144:364–367.

- Herbal medicine product name (incl. name of brand or extract and manufacturer)
- Characteristics of the herbal product (parts of plants, type of product, concentration)
- Dosage regimen and quantitative description (contents, dosage and time of intervention)
- Practitioner (training and practice experience)

Homeopathy

Reporting Data on Homeopathic Treatments (RedHot): A Supplement to CONSORT. THE JOURNAL OF ALTERNATIVE AND COMPLEMENTARY MEDICINE Volume 13, Number 1, 2007, pp. 19–23 DOI: 10.1089/acm.2006.6352

- Type of homeopathy (individualized, clinical homeopathy, isopathy or complex homeopathy)
- Type of medication (remedies, manufacturer, dilution, dosage)
- Consultations (duration, frequency)
- Qualification of practitioners (homeopathy style, training and experience)

Step 2: Define your control

The control intervention is also predefined by your study question. However, there are many details which still need to be clarified. You can have more than one control group, for example a placebo control group and a no treatment control group.

If you plan a placebo controlled trial you have to develop a placebo control group for the study. Keep in mind the placebo should be indistinguishable from the study intervention. For example for acupuncture the form of sham acupuncture (penetrating or non-penetrating) and the needling details (point location, number of needles, depths, stimulation, needle retention time, needle type) have to be defined. If you plan a trial on herbal medicine you have to choose the application form (e.g. capsule, tincture, powder) and you should ensure that appearance and smell are similar to the study intervention. A placebo for homeopathic medicines is less complicated, but you have to decide how the placebo is manufactured.

If you use a standard treatment control you should ensure that it reflects the current standard treatment for this disease. If treatment guidelines are available you should adhere to them when you design your control intervention.

If you decide to use a no-treatment control you should be sure that this is possible and will not cause any ethical problems. In addition, you should offer the patients in this control group treatment at the end of the waiting time. This will motivate them to participate and stay in the study.

When you plan a usual care control you should ensure that the care definitely reflects usual care. Standardization does not matter for this kind of control. When choosing your study centers you have to allow heterogeneity to reflect routine medical care. In addition a larger sample size is very helpful.

Step 3: Define your co-interventions

After defining your intervention and control you should think about possible co-interventions. For example if you use a placebo control in a pain study you have to allow a rescue medication for ethical purposes. In efficacy studies you should clearly define the drugs and the maximum dosage allowed. In addition the intake should be documented e.g. in a diary and reported as secondary outcome.

If you are planning a pragmatic clinical trial in usual care you might allow more heterogeneous co-interventions (e.g. all patients are allowed to use usual care in addition to the study intervention). In this kind of trial it is necessary that you have proper documentation of the co-interventions e.g. by asking patients about these details in the follow-up questionnaires.

4.3.3 Case studies

Case study 1: Uncontrolled observational study (pilot study)

Case study 1 is a descriptive, observational study without control group evaluating a treatment with special acupuncture needles that are left in situ for 7 days, an uncommon procedure but one frequently used by a particular acupuncturist.

Step 1: Define your study intervention

The intervention follows the protocol which is used by Andrew for his usual patients. According to this protocol patients receive one session with retained needles. The acupuncture points are chosen according to the Chinese medicine pattern diagnosis and the needles are left in place for 7 days.

Step 2: Define your control intervention

This is an observational study with a pre-post-comparison which has no control group.

Step 3: Define your co-interventions

This study has an observational nature and the study participants are recruited from Andrew's usual patients. Co-interventions cannot be prohibited, but are documented during the study.

Case study 2: Randomized double-blind placebo-controlled study

Case study 2 is an efficacy study. The objective of this randomized controlled trial is to evaluate whether an herbal medicine product containing an extract of Harpagophytum procumbens (Devil's claw) and given for two months is more effective than placebo in patients with chronic low back pain.

Step 1: Define your study intervention

The treatment protocol for the Devil's claw group is based on a literature search and a consensus process including 10 members of the International Society of Phytomedicine. Patients receive 1,500 mg (1 coated tablet of 750 mg two times per day) of a dried alcoholic extract from Harpagophytum procumbens over 2 months.

Step 2: Define your control intervention

The placebo is developed by the company that produces the herbal intervention. Patients receive 1 coated tablet with the same appearance as the verum intervention twice per day over 2 months.

Step 3: Define your co-interventions

Patients are allowed to treat chronic low back pain with oral non-steroidal anti-inflammatory drugs, whenever required. However the use of corticosteroids or pain-relieving drugs that act through the central nervous system is prohibited. Co-interventions are documented in a diary.

Case study 3: Pragmatic randomized study comparing three groups

Case study 3 is a comparative effectiveness study in a usual care setting. The objective of this pragmatic, randomized, three-armed trial is to evaluate whether acupuncture treatment or yoga given in addition to usual care is more effective than usual care alone for the treatment of patients with chronic low back pain and whether one of these treatments is more effective than the other.

Step 1: Define your study intervention

Intervention 1 is individualised needle acupuncture lasting 20–30 minutes per treatment; up to 12 sessions within 3 months are provided. The number of needles and the location of the acupuncture points are fully individualised and reflect usual care.

Intervention 2 consists of 12 Viniyoga sessions (90 min per session, one session per week, following the curriculum of the respective centers) within 3 months, in addition to usual care

Step 2: Define your control intervention

The control intervention is usual conventional care which should reflect the medical care patients usually receive without further standardisation of the treatment.

Step 3: Define your co-interventions

Both intervention groups will be allowed to receive usual care. Patients in the control group receive neither acupuncture nor yoga.

REFERENCES

Walach H, Haeusler W, Lowes T, Mussbach D, Schamell U, Springer W et al. Classical homeopathic treatment of chronic headaches. Cephalalgia 1997;17:119–26.

Watanabe K, Matsuura K, Gao P, Hottenbacher L, Tokunaga H, Nishimura K, Imazu Y, Reissenweber H, Witt CM. Traditional Japanese kampo medicine: clinical research between modernity and traditional medicine – the state of research and methodological suggestions for the future. eCAM 2011; doi:10.1093/ecam/neq067.

4.4 Randomization

This chapter provides information for the planning and implementation of appropriate randomization in your study.

4.4.1 Individual and cluster randomization

In every trial with more than one group, the most fundamental issue is how the groups are formed. **Randomization** is the best method to ensure a fair comparison. The principle of randomization has been described in ➢ chapter 2.

Randomization of individual patients is the most frequent approach, and almost all drug studies and efficacy studies are done in that way. However, in some situations it may be necessary or preferable to randomly assign so-called clusters of individuals (such as families, medical practices, clinics, etc.) rather than individuals. This is typically the case when the intervention is done at the cluster level. For example, in the early evaluation of mammography for breast cancer screening, some studies randomized counties: screening was offered in half of the counties, but not in the other half. Another example would be evaluation of an educational intervention for management of depression. This could be implemented in half of the participating family medicine practices but not in the other half. This type of randomization is called cluster randomization (Campbell et al. 2004). However, note that cluster randomization is associated with several problems. A statistical problem is that the outcomes of the patients in a cluster cannot be considered as independent. A methodological problem is that concealment (see below) is often difficult in cluster-randomized trials. Cluster randomization should thus only be used if there are convincing arguments, e.g. if it is the only way to organize the trial with the resources available, and preference should be given to randomizing patients.

Although randomization is the most crucial step in randomized trials it is often executed and reported poorly (Moher et al. 2010). It has been shown that inadequate randomization is associated with overly positive findings (Schulz et al. 1995). If you use random allocation in your trial you must make sure that the whole process is performed properly.

4

4.4.2 Practical steps

Randomization process	
Step 1	Make sure your allocation is concealed.
Step 2	How will you generate the randomization sequence?
Step 3	Allocate to groups at equal or unequal ratios
Step 4	Simple or restricted randomization?
Step 5	Implement the randomization process

4

Step 1: Make sure your allocation is concealed

The most important issue when allocating study participants to groups is allocation concealment. This implies two things: 1) the study personnel must be unable to predict the group to which a participant will be allocated until the patient is definitely included and registered for the study. 2) After allocation this group status must not be modified (except for well-documented compelling medical, ethical or other reasons).

Empirical investigations have shown that concealment is the most critical element of the allocation process (Schulz et al., 1995). In double-blind trials of drug treatments, concealment is usually straightforward: a manufacturer or a pharmacist who has the randomization lists prepares identically packaged, consecutively numbered drug containers (➤ Table 4.2). The researchers do not know which containers contain the studied drug and which the placebo or comparison drug. They simply give out the medication packages consecutively. The code is only broken after the study has been completed and the database "frozen".

In non-drug trials the situation is considerably more difficult. Depending on resources and logistics there are two main possibilities. One is typically described as "central randomization". Most often this means that after including a patient the researcher contacts an external clinical trial or statistics unit, although randomization tools from the internet are used increasingly. There the patient must be registered unambiguously as included in the trial. After that the person at the trial or statistics unit informs the researcher by phone or fax about the allocation status. Another approach is to use two separate databases (Vickers, 2006) avoiding the need for a separate trial unit. In one database, which is accessible to the clinicians, new patients are registered. After the registration the information is sent to a separate database, which is password protected and can only accessed by an independent person, where the randomization takes place. The information about group status is then sent back to the clinician. This method avoids clinicians arguing about allocation with staff at the clinical trial unit. Indeed, we have experienced cases of well-meaning physicians trying to have patients "re-allocated" to the group which they considered more appropriate.

Table 4.2 Frequently used, suitable methods for concealment

Concealment method	Area of use	Advantages (+)/ drawbacks (–)
Consecutively numbered drug containers	Drug trials	+ straightforward – possible only in drug trials
Central phone or fax randomization	All trials (mostly non-drug trials)	+ well accepted – costs; not absolutely foolproof
Central randomization with separate databases	All trials (mostly non-drug trials)	+ foolproof – not always available
Sequentially, numbered, opaque, sealed envelopes	All non-drug trials	+ almost always possible, cheap – cheap; has been abused in the past

The most widespread solution in "low-budget" non-drug studies is the use of sequentially numbered, opaque, sealed envelopes (SNOSE; ➤ Fig. 4.3). Each of these envelopes contains a sheet of paper designating the group allocation of a single patient. The production of these envelopes involves, as a first step, the generation of a random number list defining the sequence of group allocation. Group allocations are then written on single sheets of paper which are sealed in consecutively numbered envelopes strictly following the random number list initially produced. This simple method is straightfor-

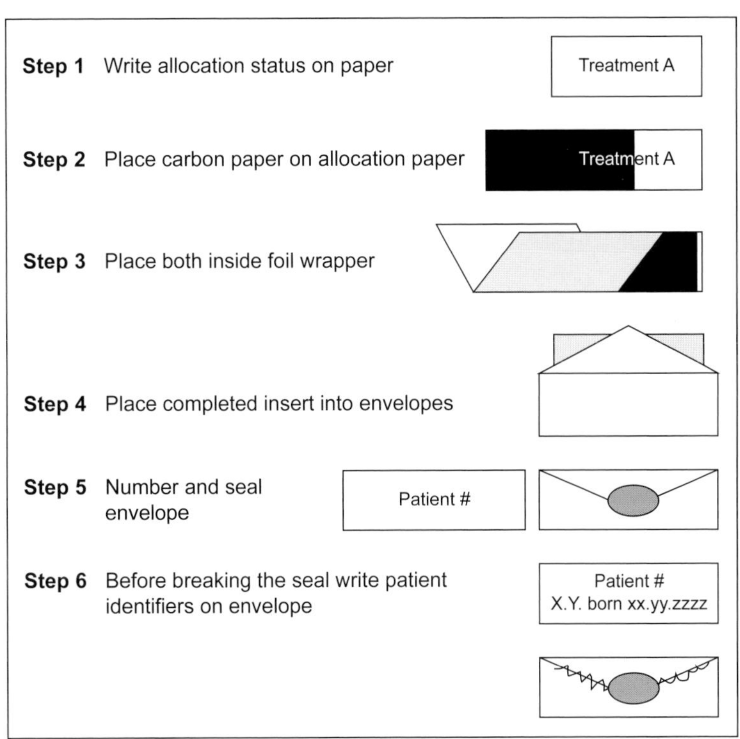

Fig. 4.3 Adequate concealment using sealed envelopes

ward, but there are documented cases where the allocation became unconcealed (Schulz, 1995). If you want to make sure that your procedure is accepted you should take particular safeguards, e.g making sure that the envelopes you use are truly opaque. For example, you can use silver foil so that a researcher cannot use a light source to see what is written inside the envelope (Doig and Simpson, 2005). Another safeguard is putting a carbon paper into the envelope. Before opening the envelope identifying information of the newly included patient is written on the envelope. Because of the carbon paper, this information becomes visible on the allocation sheet. This safeguard ensures that envelopes are not re-used or discarded if the allocation for a given patient does not seem satisfactory. In modern times the use of SNOSE seems antiquated, but in many situations it is the easiest way. An excellent description of how to implement SNOSE, also for restricted randomization etc., is provided by Doig and Simpson (2005). We also strongly recommend separating tasks whenever possible: for example, SNOSE should be kept by a person not otherwise involved in the study.

This emphasis on concealment may seem a bit obsessive – but it is clearly the most important step where selection bias can and has to be prevented. So if you randomize, you must take care that your concealment will be considered adequate (➢ Table 4.2)!

Step 2: How will you generate the randomization sequence?

Another important decision (to be taken with your statistician) is how you actually generate the randomization sequence. In principle, there are many ways to generate a random sequence (Jadad and Enkin, 2007). The most basic methods are flipping a coin or throwing a dice. Older statistics textbook typically contain tables with random numbers in their appendices. Using these researchers created a grouping sequence, for example by consecutively coding uneven numbers for group A and even numbers for group B. However, these methods should not be used any more.

The randomization sequence should be generated with suitable computer software.
A plethora of commercial and freely available software programs are available for generating random sequences. MS EXCEL also allows the creation of pseudo-random numbers which can be used to prepare allocation sequences. Professional statistical software such as SAS, SPSS or Stata include tools to generate random lists. Freeware for generating randomization sequences include EpiCalc, Random, etc. Most software programs produce pseudo-random numbers instead of true random sequences but this is usually not a problem in clinical research.

While, in principle, you can easily generate a random sequence yourself it is always good to have a statistician involved in this step. He/she will probably know adequate tools to generate the sequence. This also ensures that the function of generating the allocation sequence is separated from other functions such as coordination of the study or inclusion of patients.

You should discuss with the statistician whether the allocation sequence should be generated before the study (and recorded on one or several lists held at a secure place) or whether the sequence generation should take place whenever a new patient is included. The choice of process will depend on the following steps (particularly step 4).

If you decide to randomize you have to use a proper procedure allowing adequate concealment. Do **not** use quasi-random methods such as alternation (for example, patient one receives treatment A, patient two receives treatment B), allocation based on date of birth (for example, patients with an even birthday receive treatment A, those with an odd birthday treatment B) or day of admission (for example, patients admitted on a Monday receive treatment A, patients admitted on a Tuesday treatment B). The main problem with these methods is that the person deciding whether a patient is included in a trial knows in advance which treatment a patient will receive. If you use such an insecure method your randomization will not be considered adequate!

Step 3: Allocate to the groups in equal or unequal ratios?

As a third step you should decide whether patients will be allocated to the groups in **equal** or **unequal** numbers.

In a two-armed trial patients are normally randomized in an **equal** ratio 1 : 1, that is that the probability of a patient being randomized to the experimental or to the control group is the same, which in the majority of cases results in similar numbers of patients in the two groups. If you design a three or four armed trial the usual ratio would be 1 : 1 : 1 (each patient has 33 % chance of ending up in a given group) or 1 : 1 : 1 : 1 (25 %).

However, there can be situations in which **unequal randomization** is preferable. For example, in research on depression a new drug is sometimes tested simultaneously against a proven drug and a placebo. For ethical reasons it may be preferable to randomize only a smaller proportion of patients to placebo. Furthermore, for statistical reasons you need fewer patients for showing that the new drug is superior to placebo than for showing equivalence (or non-inferiority) of the new and the old drug. For example, a 2 : 2 : 1 ratio was used in a trial comparing a hypericum extract, imipramine and placebo (Philipp et al. 1999). However, unequal randomization has several disadvantages (loss of statistical power, consequences for blocking, difficulties with blinding of the statistician), and should only be used if there are important reasons for doing so.

Step 4: Simple or restricted randomization?

If you run a small trial and simply randomize patients to an experimental and a control group there is a considerable risk that your groups will differ at baseline just by chance. Therefore, in a third step you should decide whether you want to use simple randomization or restricted randomization (Moher et al. 2010).

Simple randomization means that there is a single sequence of random assignments. Patients are randomized regardless of their characteristics or where they are recruited, and how many patients have been allocated to a given group before. This can result in imbalances, particularly in small trials, that are materially relevant. For example, in a 40-patient trial, there is a 15 % chance that simple randomization will result in an imbalance with 25 or more patients in one group and 15 or less in the other (Vickers 2006). Similarly, there can be differences in relevant baseline characteristics.

Such problems can be prevented by using **restricted randomization**. Restricted randomization is any procedure to control the randomization to achieve balance between groups in size or characteristics. The three important methods here are blocking, stratification and minimization:

- **Blocking** or **blocked randomization** is used to ensure that the number of patients in the groups is similar. If in a two-armed trial with a randomization ratio of 1 : 1 the block size is 4, this means that among the first 4 patients 2 will be randomized to the experimental and 2 to the control group (➢ Fig. 4.4).
  One important problem with blocked randomization is that allocation becomes predictable in some patients. If staff recruiting patients know the block size and see that 2 patients have been randomized to control, they will know that the next 2 will be allocated to the experimental group. Therefore, the block size must not be told to staff recruiting the patients.
  Nevertheless, whenever possible you should use variable block sizes (for example, 2, 4, 6, 8 or 10) in a random order. If you use a suitable computer program for randomization, you first enter the various block sizes, then the program will randomly choose one of those, and only after that generate the allocation sequence. This is called **permuted block design**.
- **Stratification** or **stratified randomization** is used to ensure that groups are similar for important characteristics. Patients who share a defined characteristic are randomized separately. For example, in a trial on patients with heart failure it would be advisable to stratify for severity. You would first check whether a patient has mild to moderate disease (NYHA classification I to II) or more severe disease (NYHA III), and then proceed with separate randomization for these "strata".
  In multicenter trials the single centers are often separate strata (➢ Fig. 4.4). Since patients included in a study as well as their prognoses might differ in different practices or hospitals, it is important that similar numbers of patients are allocated to the experimental treatment or to the control condition in each study center.
  To make sure that stratification is efficient it is better to use blocking within strata (Moher et al. 2010).
- Be very careful when deciding on blocking and stratification. For example, if you stratify for three factors (age > 65 or not, gender, NYHA I, II or III) there are 12 possible strata combinations (2 for age × 2 for gender × 3 for the 3 NYHA classes). It is very likely that there will be very small numbers of patients for some of these combinations and your whole exercise becomes counter-productive.

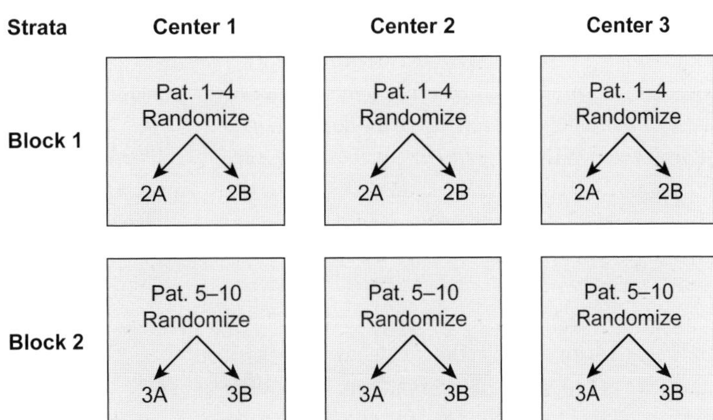

Fig. 4.4 Block randomization stratified by center

- **Minimization** is a technique which tries to ensure that the groups are comparable for several factors. In this case randomization lists cannot be prepared in advance (see Step 1). Minimization is not a true random allocation technique but accepted as a valid alternative (Moher et al., 2010). It takes account of the characteristics of patients included so far and modifies the probabilities of a new patient with defined characteristics of being allocated to a given group. The process usually also includes a random component. If you consider using minmization in your trial you have to discuss and plan this in detail with a competent statistician.

Step 5: Implement the randomization process

In the final step you should plan how you implement the randomization process in reality. Who does what, and when? Reconsider whether the planned strategy is feasible and efficient. Then write it up carefully as a standard operating procedure (SOP, ➢ Ch. 5). If you are accurate here it will be no problem for you to provide a good description of your randomization method in the publication of your trial.

4.4.3 Case studies

Case study 1: Uncontrolled observational study (pilot study)

Case study 1 is a descriptive, observational study without control group evaluating a treatment with special acupuncture needles that are left in situ for 7 days – an uncommon procedure but one frequently used by a particular acupuncturist: randomization is not performed in this study.

Case study 2: Randomized double-blind placebo-controlled study

Case study 2 is an efficacy study which is performed within the appropriate regulatory framework. The objective of this randomized controlled trial is to evaluate whether Devil's claw is more effective than placebo after two months' treatment of patients with chronic low back pain.

Step 1: Make sure your allocation is concealed

Identically packaged, consecutively numbered drug containers will be used to ensure concealed randomization.

Step 2: How will you create a proper randomization sequence?

A statistician creates the randomization list using a computer program.

Step 3: Allocate to groups at equal or unequal ratios?

Since in this trial there is no specific reason why patients should be allocated in an unequal ratio, patients will be allocated in the ratio 1 : 1.

Step 4: Simple or restricted randomization?

Randomization should be done stratified by center and using a permuted block design.

Step 5: Implement the randomization process

The manufacturer will receive a randomization list from the statistician. According to this list the manufacturer prepares identically packaged, consecutively numbered drug containers. With the exception of the person responsible for packaging, nobody knows which containers contain the studied drug and which placebo. Providers simply give out the medication packages consecutively after including patients. The code will only be revealed after the study is completed (except in cases of emergency when it is necessary to reveal the code for an individual patient, ➢ Ch. 4.6).

Case study 3: Pragmatic randomized study comparing three groups

Case study 3 is a comparative effectiveness study in a usual care setting. The objective of this pragmatic, randomized, three-armed trial is to evaluate whether acupuncture treatment or yoga given in addition to usual care is more effective than usual care alone in the management of patients with chronic low back pain and whether acupuncture is more effective than yoga in this context.

Step 1: Make sure your allocation is concealed

Central telephone randomization will be used to ensure allocation concealment.

Step 2: How will you create a proper randomization sequence?

A statistician creates the randomization list using a computer program.

Step 3: Allocate to groups at equal or unequal ratios?

Since in this trial there is no specific reason why patients should be allocated in an unequal ratio, patients will be allocated in the ratio 1 : 1 : 1.

Step 4: Simple or restricted randomization?

Randomization should be done stratified by recruiting center and using a permuted block design.

Step 5: Implement the randomization process

Once a patient has been included into the study, the relevant study centre (a general practice) faxes the details of the newly included person (name, date of birth, participant and centre codes, date of inclusion) and a copy of the signed informed consent form to the central randomization unit at an independent statistics institute. Then the study centre calls the randomization unit and confirms the information which is entered into a database. After this information has been saved the database will show the group that this patient is allocated to. The staff member from the randomization unit tells the centre the allocation and sends a fax for confirmation. If the patient is allocated to the acupuncture group he/she is referred to an acupuncture practice, if randomized to the Viniyoga group he/she is referred to a local yoga centre.

REFERENCES

Campbell MK, Elbourne DR, Altman DG. CONSORT statement: extension to cluster randomised trials. *BMJ* 2004;328:7,028.

Doig GS, Simpson F. Randomization and allocation concealment: a practical guide to researchers. J Crit Care 2005;20:187–91.

Jadad A, Enkin MW. Randomised controlled trials. 2nd edition. London: Blackwell BMJ Books, 2007.

Moher D, Hopewell S, Schulz KF, Montori V, Gøtzsche PC, Devereaux PJ, Elbourne D, Egger M, Altman DG. CONSORT 2010 Explanation and Elaboration: updated guidelines for reporting parallel group randomised trials. *BMJ* 2010;340:c869. doi: 10.1136/bmj.c869. (available freely at www.consort-statement.org/consort-statement; accessed June 3, 2010)

Philipp M, Kohnen R, Hiller KO. Hypericum extract versus imipramine or placebo in patients with moderate depression: randomised multicentre study of treatment for eight weeks. *BMJ* 1999;319:1,534–8.

Schulz KF, Chalmers I, Hayes RJ, Altman DG. Empirical evidence of bias. Dimensions of methodological quality associated with estimates of treatment effects in controlled trials JAMA 1995;273:408–12.

Schulz KF. Subverting randomization in controlled trials. JAMA 1995;274:1,456–8.

Vickers AJ. How to randomize. J Soc Integrat Oncol 2006;4:194–8.

4.5 What to do if you do not randomize

This chapter provides information how differences between groups can be minimized or taken into account when allocation to groups is not randomized.

4.5.1 Taking baseline differences into account

In chapter 2 we discussed broadly the cases in which studies with a non-randomized comparison group may be appropriate. The main problem in such studies is that there are almost inevitably baseline differences between the groups at inclusion. The two main strategies to deal with differences between patients are (1) matching and (2) performing statistical analyses which adjust for imbalances between groups regarding relevant factors (confounders) that may influence the study outcome.

As we stated in ➤ chapter 2, matching is often inefficient and one has to know which prognostic factors are truly predictive of the outcome. Therefore, whenever feasible we recommend performing a parallel prospective observational study adjusting for baseline differences and other confounders in the analysis. Nevertheless since in some situations matching is the only choice we also describe this method below.

4.5.2 Matching – practical steps

Steps in a matching process	
Step 1	Select matching criteria
Step 2	Plan the matching procedure
Step 3	Test feasibility

Step 1: Select matching criteria

The matching criteria should be a) relevant with regards to prognosis, b) easy to measure, and c) not too numerous. You should review the available literature carefully for the condition of interest in order to identify potentially relevant variables. Epidemiological studies (mainly cohort studies but also case-control studies) are likely to be most helpful here since if they are done properly they carefully take confounding factors into account. Check the variables typically included in the analyses of these studies. Randomized trials are not very helpful since randomization considerably reduces the issue of confounding. Of course you should also talk to clinicians who are experts in the condition of interest.

Very often age and gender are included as matching criteria. They are easy to measure and often influence outcomes. However in order to find enough matching patients, age does not need to be identical but instead may fall into a given age window (for example, three years). If a classification into grades of severity exists for the condition investigated, this may be included as a criterion. For example, in a pair of patients with heart failure the grading according to NYHA (New York Heart Association) should be the same. Other frequently used matching criteria include treatments received so far, and time since diagnosis. The number of matching criteria is a matter of compromise. If only two or three criteria are chosen it should be relatively easy to identify plenty of matching patients in a population but the risk that patients differ in important prognostic factors is probably still considerable. If ten criteria are used, differences will be less likely but only a small number of matching pairs will probably be identified.

Step 2: Plan the matching procedure

Once you have established the matching criteria you have to decide by whom and how the matching will be done. You may be fortunate to have access to a large, well-organized database containing all relevant matching criteria (reliably coded). In that case you can let the computer search for matching patients. This not only reduces the workload but also decreases the likelihood that the process may be biased. In many situations, however, the database will not include all relevant information and thus the data will need to be supplemented by going through patients' case histories. Even worse, you may first have to collect all the data needed, either retrospectively from the case histories or prospectively in your study. Measures to reduce the possibility of bias in the process of selecting matching pairs should be implemented, such as having two reviewers independently assessing whether matching criteria are fulfilled. Unfortunately, these steps will increase the workload.

It should be kept in mind that it is not necessary to only compare *pairs*. Case-control studies in epidemiology often have up to five matching controls for one case. This increases the statistical power of the analyses.

Step 3: Test feasibility

Before starting with a large study using matching you should test whether your procedure is feasible. It might be that there is one criterion which substantially reduces the number of matching pairs. Also, you may find on clinical review that the individuals of a matched pair have quite different prognoses, even though they seemed similar according to your criteria. This could be due to a factor not included in your predefined criteria.

4.5.3 Adjusting analyses for imbalances – practical steps

Adjusting analyses for imbalances	
Step 1	Make sure your statistician is competent
Step 2	Identify potentially relevant prognostic variables/confounders
Step 3	Make sure you measure the appropriate variables
Step 4	Plan the analysis

Step 1: Make sure your statistician is competent

It is always preferable to work with a good statistician, but if you do a non-randomized controlled study in which you plan to adjust for multiple potentially confounding variables a good statistician is absolutely fundamental. While you can do a lot of basic statistical analyses in a randomized trial or an uncontrolled study yourself, the level of complexity in statistical analyses here requires a true expert. Try to find out whether your statistician has already done similar studies. You might search PubMed to check what studies he/she has done previously and you should consider contacting other statisticians to hear their opinion.

Step 2: Identify potentially relevant prognostic variables/confounders

This step resembles step 1 in the matching section. Here again you should review the literature and ask expert clinicians about the factors to be used in your study. However, as we will discuss below, this step is not as important as in studies using matching as you can (and probably will) modify the selection of variables to be included at the analysis stage.

4

Step 3: Make sure you measure the appropriate variables

In our view, a main shortcoming of many non-randomized comparative studies is the insufficient characterization of participants. If it is not possible to randomize patients, it is likely that groups will differ in various characteristics. Consider whether issues such as attitudes, beliefs, expectations, education, socioeconomic status, previous treatments, etc. may be different between groups and may affect outcomes. For a valid interpretation it is mandatory to explore and document potentially relevant differences in as much detail as possible.

Step 4: Plan the analysis

One of the advantages of adjusting for baseline differences and confounders in the analysis is that you can also include variables based on your actual findings. For example, you may find that your groups fundamentally differ a priori in a variable (e.g. educational level) that is documented but had not been considered. It is possible to check whether a variable is associated with the outcome and whether baseline values for a variable differ. When planning your study you should discuss with your statistician the broad strategy for selecting covariates for the multivariate analysis. Typically, some factors known to be important such as age, gender or baseline values of the main outcome measure are predefined as potentially relevant variables. Other factors may be selected based on significant differences detected during early analysis and their association with outcomes. Unless you have sufficient expertise you will have to rely considerably on your statistician for this step, but you should try to understand what he/she is planning to do.

4.5.4 Case study

Adapted case study 3: Non-randomized study comparing acupuncture and yoga

Our case study 3 is a comparative effectiveness study in a usual care setting. The objective of this pragmatic randomized three-armed trial is to evaluate whether acupuncture or yoga in addition to usual care is more effective than usual care alone in the treatment of patients with chronic low back pain and whether added acupuncture is more effective than added yoga. As this study is randomized the issues discussed in this chapter do not apply. Therefore, we discuss a modified study:

Imagine that instead of a randomized three-armed trial a non-randomized study comparing acupuncture and yoga is planned. You work with the acupuncture practices and the yoga centers offering classes routinely to patients suffering from chronic low back pain. As in the randomized trial, the (individualized) treatments are documented and outcomes measured after 2, 6 and 12 months in all patients who meet defined inclusion criteria. Since the study is not randomized, potential differences between outcomes will be difficult to interpret. You should thus make sure that your study provides appropriate information on other potentially confounding aspects. For example, why patients get one or other treatment, how treatment processes differ or how patients experience the different treatments. A matched-case approach does not seem appropriate here but a careful study with an analysis adjusting for baseline differences between the groups may be interesting.

Step 1: Make sure your statistician is competent

Step 2: Identify potential variables/ confounders

Search the literature for epidemiological studies in the area of low back pain and check which factors are typically relevant to prognosis. Discuss with experienced clinicians what they consider important. The literature search and the discussions may identify the following important prognostic factors: baseline levels of pain, depressive symptoms, level of activity, expectations, duration of symptoms. However, quite a number of additional factors may only be associated with preference for acupuncture and Yoga (e.g. cultural characteristics or attitudes).

Step 3: Make sure you measure the relevant baseline variables

Try to measure the factors identified in step 2 as accurately as possible. Use validated and widely used methods or instruments whenever possible.

Step 4: Plan the analysis

Discuss with your statistician which analyses are feasible and most promising. Decide on strategies to identify further potential confounders from your data.

4.6 Blinding

In this chapter we explain how to proceed if you want to implement blinding in your study.

4.6.1 Should you go for blinding?

There are many ways in which biases that occur during the study process (after allocation and before analyses) can distort study findings in open (non-blinded) studies.

If patients know which treatment they receive they may feel different, rate outcomes differently or seek other co-interventions. Without blinding, treatment providers may apply the treatments in a different manner, add different co-interventions and also rate outcomes differently. During the analysis statisticians might choose slightly different methods which sometimes can have considerable impact on the conclusions of a trial. Blinding is a crucial measure to reduce such biases.

In a controlled study there are several groups of people (or functions) for whom blinding can be considered:

- Patients/study participants
- Treatment providers
- Outcome evaluators (if not identical with patients or providers)/data collectors
- Principal investigator/trial coordinators
- Study monitors
- Data managers
- Decisions makers on inclusion in analysis populations
- Statisticians

Trials in which patients and providers are blinded are typically called **double-blind**, but this term has also been used for trials in which patients and outcome evaluators, but not providers, were blinded. If you read in the literature about a triple- or quadruple-blinded trial researchers counted each function separately, but this confusing terminology is not advocated. In principle, it is always desirable to blind as many of the parties involved in a trial as possible. Blinding is of particular relevance if outcomes are subject to reporting bias.

Patients can only be blinded

- if either a placebo or sham intervention is used in the control group;
- or if two true treatments are compared which cannot be distinguished easily (for example, two homeopathic remedies),
- or if a double dummy technique can be used.

An example where the **double dummy technique** is applied is described in the following; a study is set up to compare acupuncture with a drug treatment. One group of patients receives true acupuncture and placebo drug while the other patient group receives sham acupuncture and the true drug. The double-dummy technique allows blinding where experimental treatments are clearly distinguishable but placebos or sham techniques are available for both. Boutron et al. have provided informative overviews which methods have previously been used for blinding in both pharmacological (2006) and non-pharmacological trials (2007).

Treatment providers can be blinded easily in drug trials but almost never in non-drug trials. Even if patients and providers cannot be blinded it is sometimes possible to involve an independent person who is unaware of treatment allocation and who can assess outcomes. If this is possible, it is clearly a desirable option. However, in many areas where CAM treatments are used, the most relevant outcomes (such as pain, function or quality of life) are best assessed by the patients themselves. The resources needed for having an independent outcome evaluator, which are often considerable, make sense only if the outcome assessed by the independent evaluator is truly clinically relevant. In some cases it may be possible to blind data collection. For example, telephone interviewers contacting and interviewing patients do not have to know allocation status.

While in small trials the same person can be treatment provider, principal investigator (the person who formally has the main responsibility for the study and, hopefully, also invested most thought in it) as well as trial coordinator (the person who is responsible for the actual performance of the trial), these functions tend to be separated in large multicenter trials. If the treatment is separated from data collection and evaluation, the latter two processes may be blinded even in trials in which patients and providers are unblinded.

Study monitoring and data management are two further key functions in a controlled trial. Monitors check whether the case report forms are adequately filled in and whether procedures are performed according to the study protocol. Data managers are responsible for the data entry, take care of the database and prepare files for analysis. Whenever possible, these people (or functions, as in small trials one person might be responsible for almost everything) should also be blinded to the allocation status.

An extremely important decision is which patients should be included in the treat analysis, i. e. which patients violated the protocol seriously and so should be excluded from the per protocol analysis. It is likely that in the past the findings of a considerable number of trials have been biased because they excluded patients selectively from the analysis. Thus, it is now considered fundamental that the decision who should be included in the different analysis populations (> Ch. 6) is made under blind conditions. This can be achieved relatively easy by leaving this decision to an independent expert who is not otherwise involved in the study and unaware of the allocation status. Blinding of this part of the process can be achieved even in otherwise non-blinded trials.

Sometimes statisticians can be blinded, too. In these cases they receive only coded information (for example A and B), but are not informed which is the experimental and which the control group.

While from a methodological point of view blinding is always desirable to increase internal validity, there can be a variety of reasons for deciding against it. For example, sham procedures might act on the same physiological mechanisms as true treatment (this has been claimed in case of sham acupuncture or sham chiropractic manipulation). There may be no adequate placebo that allows successful blinding. For example, mistletoe injections are typically associated with specific erythemas and an experienced physician will clearly know whether a patient received verum or placebo. The blinding process may interfere with the normal treatment process. For example, classical homeopaths treating a patient with a chronic disease say that they often need to try out several remedies before making the correct choice. If in a placebo-controlled trial the homeopath does not know whether a patient received the true remedy or placebo, he or she does not know whether the lack of a response is due to an incorrect remedy choice or the fact that the patient was on placebo. If a trial aims to evaluate the "overall" effect of an intervention the introduction of blinding might modify the whole setting in a manner which is biasing in itself. In any case, if you choose not to employ blinding, you must be aware that the internal validity of your findings can, and probably will, be criticized. If you go for blinding, you have to plan carefully how to do it best.

4.6.2 Practical steps

Practical steps when blinding	
Step 1	Check the literature for what others have done
Step 2	Decide who can and will be blinded in your study
Step 3	Define the methods for implementing blinding
Step 4	Decide how to inform patients
Step 5	Consider pilot testing
Step 6	Prepare emergency envelopes
Step 7	Test whether blinding was successful

Step 1: Check the literature for what others have done

As for most other parts in the study protocol, you should review the literature carefully and assess how other researchers dealt with blinding, what methods were used, and what problems occurred. This point is less important for a trial of a drug without specific side effects for which an identically looking, smelling and tasting placebo can easily be prepared. But even with many herbal medicines, producing an indistinguishable and at the same time inert (or certainly not effective for the condition being treated) placebo is far from easy. In the literature you might find that other researchers have already developed a good placebo which you could use. In trials of non-drug interventions blinding is never easy. For acupuncture, osteopathy or chiropractic a variety of sham interventions have been used. Those which are very similar to the true treatment are unlikely to be physiologically inert and those which are likely to be inert may easily be detected as sham.

Step 2: Decide who can and will be blinded in your study

Based on your research question, your participants and their conditions, the interventions, the setting, your outcome and the available resources, you can now decide who could and should be blinded in your trial.

Step 3: Define the methods for implementing blinding

In trials comparing a drug with a placebo or with another drug, the implementation of blinding is quite straightforward, and if you are collaborating with a manufacturer the preparation of the medication is most likely to be done there. Still, you should know the important points to make sure the manufacturer does it well. If you use a placebo you have to decide on its composition and the measures to make it as indistinguishable from the true drug as possible. If you compare two drugs it might happen that one comes as a capsule and one as a tablet. You have to discuss with experts whether it might be possible to re-configure one to get both in the same galenic form, or whether you have to use the double-dummy technique. The test medication has to be labelled and packaged appropriately. Take care that relevant guidelines from drug regulatory agencies are taken into account. While it is open to discussion whether the statistician has to be blinded, you should make sure that all other functions mentioned above remain blinded as long as possible.

In non-drug trial things tend to be much more complicated. Based on your literature review, and your research question, etc. you choose your intervention for the control group, for example a sham acupuncture with superficial insertion of thin needles at a semistandardised selection of points some distance from true points. Your acupuncturists obviously know what they are doing. If you want to make sure that blinding is maintained, acupuncturists must not provide any clues to the patients. Sessions should be organized in a manner that patients from different groups do not meet. Consider instructing acupuncturists how they should respond to critical questions ("Doctor, could it be that I am in the sham group?"). Study monitors checking case report forms and data managers might discover the allocation status as acupuncturists have to document the points actually treated. Consider whether it is possible to separate forms or data to keep this group blinded. Think through the whole study, trying to figure out what problems might occur, and how they can be fixed. The issues and eventualities you have to think of will vary greatly depending on the processes in the specific trials. It is crucial that you try to think through the whole process.

Step 4: Decide how to inform patients

Each patient entering a trial has to be informed about the objectives, methods and processes in a trial. This can be a problem for blinding. If, for example, you use the sham acupuncture intervention described in step 3 and tell patients that half of them will receive acupuncture at correct points and half at "placebo" points some patients will try to find out whether "their" points can be found in acupuncture textbooks. However, if you tell patients that half receive acupuncture and half a placebo the situation might be quite different, as patients being needled might automatically consider this to be acupuncture while they would expect placebo to be something different. Some trials use information which is not fully transparent (for example: "We shall compare needling at points indicated according to traditional medicine with needling at points not selected according to this theory") or even obscuring ("We shall compare two types of acupuncture"). This enhances the likelihood that patients believe that they receive a true treatment and do not try to find out whether they are in the sham group. However, this is ethically problematic. If the theory of acupuncture is taken seriously some of the information as outlined above is clearly deceptive. In some countries such information will not pass ethical review while in others researchers may even be encouraged to use such deceptive information. You will have to carefully consider ethical and methodological implications.

Independently from the blinding issue, the way you inform patients may also influence expectations and attitudes of patients, and there is evidence indicating that this can influence outcome (Hrobjartssin & Gøtzsche 2010). In conclusion, the way you phrase the information about the treatments provided in a blinded trial can have considerable impact on blinding as well as on results.

Step 5: Consider pilot testing

Unless you use a straightforward blinding procedure or you have experience with the method used, you should consider testing whether your blinding procedure works. While a pilot study would be the optimal way to do this, you should at least test the procedure in a group of volunteers. This will give you clues to whether there are fundamental problems on a practical level.

Step 6: Prepare emergency envelopes

If you perform a trial in which the clinicians are blinded you have to be prepared for the case when an unexpected situation (for example a serious adverse event) necessitates breaking the blinding code for an individual patient. You have to decide whether you need so-called **emergency envelopes** which contain the information on the allocation status. In this case you also have to take care that these envelopes are not abused to undermine concealment or blinding.

Emergency envelopes must be sealed carefully and opaque (similarly to envelopes used for concealment of random allocation – ➢ Ch. 4.4), and have to be checked regularly. Reasons for breaking emergency envelopes have to be documented.

Step 7: Test whether blinding was successful

It is quite likely that some patients will find out their allocation status during a trial. This can bias the findings of a trial. Consequently a number of CAM researchers have in recent years tried to test whether blinding was successful, even though this is very rarely done in conventional medicine (Hróbjartsson et al. 2007). There are two main methods to do this: allocation guessing and credibility ratings.

Allocation guessing means that patients (and/or physicians) are asked what treatment they think they received (or applied, respectively). However, there are a number of problems with this approach. One problem is that there are various ways to ask for allocation guessing. You can give patients the option to choose only between the actual treatment alternatives, you can include a "don't know" option, or additionally you can ask patients how certain they are about their guess. However, the main problem is that if one intervention is clearly more effective than the other, perceived effects influence guesses. For example, a patient who experienced a clear improvement is more likely to guess that he/she received the true treatment than to guess having received placebo. Therefore, trials where true differences of effectiveness exist between experimental and control group have a priori a higher likelihood that allocation guessing will find unblinding than trials where there is no true difference. You can ask patients why they made a specific guess and this might give hints whether unblinding is due to differential effectiveness or to other factors but it is unclear how reliable such questions are. You can also consider asking patients for allocation guessing before a perceivable treatment effect is expected. However, if unblinding (whether related to effectiveness or other factors) occurs later in the trial this is not detected. Furthermore, asking patients to give allocation guesses early in the trial might motivate patients to try to find out what group they are in.

An alternative or addition to asking for allocation guesses is credibility rating. This approach was originally used in behavioral therapy (Borkovec and Nau 1972). We have had positive experiences with a modified version (Vincent 1990) in several trials of acupuncture (➢ Table 4.2). Credibility rating assesses blinding success indirectly by investigating whether participants have confidence in the actual treatment they receive. The advantage of credibility

Table 4.3 Credibility assessment by Vincent (1990; modified from Borkovec & Nau 1972). Answer options are on a scale from 0 to 6 with 0 indicating very low confidence and 6 very high confidence.

Question
1. How confident do you feel that this treatment can alleviate your complaint?
2. How confident would you be in recommending this treatment to a friend who suffered from a similar complaint?
3. How logical does this treatment seem to you?
4. In your opinion how successful may this treatment be in alleviating other complaints?

ratings is that patients are not pushed into doubt. However, in principle they suffer from the same problems as allocation guessing.

Including questions on allocation guessing and/or credibility in your study indicates that you really want to be rigorous. However, you might be causing trouble for yourself: if your trial finds a clear effect of treatment over control and you have an indication that unblinding has occured, you might have difficulty getting your trial published in a good journal.

4.6.3 Case studies

Case study 1: Uncontrolled observational study (pilot study)

Case study 1 is a descriptive, observational study without control group evaluating a treatment with special acupuncture needles that are left in situ for 7 days – an uncommon procedure but one frequently used by a particular acupuncturist – there will be no blinding in this study

Case study 2: Randomized double-blind placebo-controlled study

Case study 2 is an efficacy study which is performed within the appropriate regulatory framework. The objective of this randomized controlled trial is to evaluate whether Devil's claw is more effective than placebo after two months treatment of patients with chronic low back pain.

Step 1: Check the literature for previously used procedures

Previously published placebo-controlled trials used coated tablets without the extract. This seems a reasonable approach which is also chosen for this study.

Step 2: Decide who can and will be blinded in your study

Consider all participants/contributors: patients (who also assess the major outcomes), physicians and other carers, principal investigators, study monitors, data managers, those who decide on analysis populations and the statistician.

Step 3: Define the methods for implementing blinding

The manufacturer prepares two lots of coated tablets, with the extract and without (placebo). The tablets have exactly the same appearance and similar smell and taste. They are put into blister packs which are only opened immediately before the drug is taken. According to the randomization lists, the manufacturer prepares identically packaged, consecutively numbered drug containers. With the exception of the person responsible for packaging, nobody knows which containers contain the drug in question and which the placebo. Providers simply give out the medication packages consecutively to patients after they have been included. The code will be revealed only after the study is completed. The statistician will receive a data file giving A and B as code for treatments only.

Step 4: Decide how to inform patients

According to regulations and ethical standards patients are informed that they have a 50 : 50 chance of receiving the true treatment (Latin = verum) or placebo.

Step 5: Consider pilot testing

A formal pilot study does not seem necessary. However, we would suggest pre-testing whether verum and placebo are indistinguishable by giving them (first either verum or placebo, then, after making an assessment, the other tablets for direct comparison) both to individuals who have never taken or been prescribed Devil's claw and to some individuals who are familiar with it. If these tests reveal that verum and placebo can be distinguished easily the placebo should be developed further to make it more similar to the verum.

Step 6: Prepare emergency envelopes

Since in this study almost all people involved are blinded, emergency envelopes must be available in case of emegencies. These have to be prepared in the manner described in chapter 4.4 (consecutively numbered, sealed, opaque envelopes) and stored at a place which is both safe and always accessible. Measures have to be taken that breaking of emergenciy envelopes occurs only if necessary and is carefully documented.

Step 7: Test whether blinding was successful

Tests of blinding are not widely used for drug trials. Still, we would ask patients to fill in a credibility questionnaire after two weeks of treatment (Devil's claw is expected to have clinically relevant effects only after two to four weeks) and we would ask physicians and patients to make an allocation guess at the end of the observation period.

Case study 3: Pragmatic randomized study comparing three groups

Case study 3 is a comparative effectiveness study in a usual care setting. The objective of this pragmatic randomized three-armed trial is to evaluate whether acupuncture treatment or yoga given in addition to usual care is more effective than usual care alone in the treatment of patients with chronic low back pain and whether acupuncture treatment is more effective than yoga in this context.

Step 1: Check the literature for what others have done

Does not really apply – you will find little about blinding such trials in the literature.

Step 2: Decide who can and will be blinded in your study

We would only blind the statistical analysis of the principal outcomes in this trial.

Patients and providers cannot be blinded. As the most relevant outcome assessments are done by the patients themselves, outcome measurement will not be blinded either. Having a blinded evaluator (a clinician unaware to which group patients have been allocated) is a theoretical option but is rarely feasible. Assessments for low back pain by a clinician are not considered very important. Organising a blind assessment would need considerable resources and is logistically difficult (blinded clinician not likely to be available; need for additional participant visits; training of evaluators, etc.). We would thus recommend not having a blinded evaluation. However what may be considered is having blinded interviewers in those cases where some of the outcomes are collected via telephone interview, or collecting data blinded if, for example, insurance data, is used. Still, as these are only secondary issues in our case study we assume here that there will be no blinding on this level either. We would not blind the principal investigator and it would be difficult to blind study monitors and data managers as they will have to check the documentation on study treatments and co-interventions. Because the main analysis will use a strict intention to treat approach, blinding also has little impact on the decision of who will be in which analysis population.

Step 3: Define the methods to implement blinding

The statistician will receive a data file which includes only the letters A, B and C for the three groups without any information for which letter stands for which group.

Step 4: Decide how to inform patients

Not relevant as patients will not be blinded.

Step 5: Consider pilot testing

Not applicable

Step 6: Prepare emergency envelopes

Not necessary as key persons are not blinded

Step 7: Test whether blinding was successful

Not applicable

REFERENCES
Borkovec TD, Nau SD. Credibility of analogue therapy rationales. J Behav Ther Exp Psychiat 1972;3:257–60.
Boutron I, Estellat C, Guittet L, Dechartres A, Sackett DL, Hróbjartsson A, Ravaud P. Methods of blinding in reports of randomized controlled trials assessing pharmacologic treatments: a systematic review. PLoS Med. 2006;3:e425.
Boutron I, Guittet L, Estellat C, Moher D, Hróbjartsson A, Ravaud P. Reporting methods of blinding in randomized trials assessing nonpharmacological treatments. PLoS Med. 2007;4:e61.
Hróbjartsson A, Forfang E, Haahr MT, Als-Nielsen B, Brorson S. Blinded trials taken to the test: an analysis of randomized clinical trials that report tests for the success of blinding. Int J Epidemiol. 2007;36:654–63.
Hrobjartsson A, Gotzsche PC. Placebo interventions for all clinical conditions. Cochrane Database Syst Rev 2010;(1):CD003974.
Vincent CA. Credibility assessments in trials of acupuncture. Complement Med Res 1990;4(1):8–11.

4.7 Study participants

This chapter summarizes the issues to be considered regarding inclusion and exclusion of trial participants.

4.7.1 Who should be included in your study?

Deciding who should actually participate in your study is crucial in the planning process. "Study participant" is a neutral term that can be used for both healthy volunteers and patients. The optimal strategy for recruiting and including participants can vary considerably from study to study and depends on your study question. Factors influencing participant selection include access to patients, design aspects, ethical issues and whether you want to perform a strict efficacy or a pragmatic effectiveness trial. For example, if you want to answer a narrow efficacy question you may want to include an extremely well-defined group of patients suffering from migraine without aura, and exclude all patients who have additional tension type headache, attacks with aura, or other relevant co-morbidity. However, if you want to do a pragmatic multi-center trial to investigate whether your treatment provides clinically relevant additional benefits to routine care under routine conditions you will probably use much more liberal inclusion criteria allowing for inclusion of patients who have symptoms of a wider definition.

4.7.2 Practical steps

Steps when selecting study participants	
Step 1	Develop inclusion and exclusion criteria
Step 2	Assess access to patients
Step 3	Plan the screening and inclusion process
Step 4	Decide how to inform patients

Step 1: Develop inclusion and exclusion criteria

Every clinical study protocol should include a list of inclusion criteria (criteria that must be met for the inclusion of a patient) and exclusion criteria (issues that rule out participation). ➤ Fig. 4.5 gives an example of a typical list of inclusion and exclusion criteria. As for any other planning issue the published literature will help you greatly in defining these criteria. The method section of every study publication describes selection criteria. Once you have read a number of relevant articles you will have a collection of the most relevant points. Make sure that you take current standards for appropriate diagnostic classifications into account. For example, if you set up a trial on depression you will need to classify your participating patients according to the International Classification of Diseases (ICD, current version 10) or the Diagnostic and Statistical Manual for Mental Disorders (DSM, current version IV), otherwise your paper will not be accepted in a prestigious journal. Colleagues will want to understand the selection criteria for participants in your study. Consider whether you require a minimum severity level of symptoms for the inclusion of a patient. The advantage of this is that you only include patients in which treatment is indicated and who have a chance to improve. However, having a minimum severity might also cause problems: you will probably get some regression to the mean (➤ Ch. 2) and patients or physicians may rate severity inappropriately high to meet the inclusion criterion. So consider carefully which of these risks is more pronounced in your study. Particularly for uncontrolled studies, you might consider including only patients whose disease activity has been either stable or developing in a consistent manner. This will make the interpretation of observed changes easier. Make sure that you exclude patients whose participation could put them at risk, for example, patients who take medication that could result in dangerous interactions with your study treatment. Be aware that special ethical problems are associated with trials involving pregnant women, children, people with a limited ability to understand the study or to give informed consent, or those in situations in which free decision-making may be compromised (for example, in prisoners).

Screening-Nr.: ☐☐☐ Study centre: _☐☐☐

Checklist of inclusion and exclusion criteria

1. Age 18 to 65 years
   ☐ yes ☐ no – STOP
2. Drug-induced headache suspected/intake of drugs against headaches on more than 10 days per month
   ☐ yes – STOP ☐ no
3. Acupuncture treatment in the last 6 months
   ☐ yes – STOP ☐ no
4. Serious somatic or mental disease present
   ☐ yes – STOP ☐ no
5. Diagnosis of migraine with or without aura (ICD-10: G43.0, G43.1, G44.20/21):
   ☐ yes ☐ no – STOP
6. Migraine for at least 12 months
   ☐ yes ☐ no – STOP
7. Two to eight migraine attacks per month in the last 3 months
   ☐ yes ☐ no – STOP
8. Onset of first migraine attack after 50 years of age
   ☐ yes – STOP ☐ no
9. Migraine prophylaxis with drugs in the last 4 weeks
   ☐ yes – STOP ☐ no
10. In addition to migraine the patient also has tension-type headache on more than 10 days per month
    ☐ yes – STOP ☐ no
11. The patient suffers from additional tension-type headache and is unable to distinguish migraine from tension type headaches
    ☐ yes – STOP ☐ no

Fig. 4.5 Form for checking the most relevant inclusion and exclusion criteria in an explanatory randomized trial of acupuncture for migraine prophylaxis with narrow inclusion (modified from Linde et al. 2005)

Step 2: Assess access to patients

Even the best collection of selection criteria will not help if you have no access to potential participants. Ideally you will be working in a unit or network which has already been involved in several studies for the condition of interest and which has some idea of the number patients presenting with the relevant problem given specific inclusion criteria. Previous studies may show how many patients are likely to give consent to be randomized and how variable their symptoms will be. Unfortunately, these ideal conditions are the exception for most CAM researchers. Practitioners tend to overestimate (grossly) the number of patients that meet the eligibility criteria. So you need to consider carefully whether your study is attractive to patients or whether they can get the same treatment without being bothered by randomization and questionnaires. Try to pre-empt potential obstacles and problems for the recruitment and the selection process, and find ways these can be prevented.

Step 3: Plan the screening and inclusion process

It is now considered mandatory that the selection process of a study is well documented. Publications of clinical trials routinely include flow charts (➢ Ch. 7) which show not only the number of patients leaving a trial prematurely but also how many patients have been checked for eligibility and how many were excluded and for what reasons. This allows the reader to assess whether the participants of your study are likely to represent normal clinic patients or whether they are a highly selected (atypical) group.

!

For your study, this means that you should carefully document all contacts including those which do not result in inclusion into the study.
Some of the reasons for non-inclusion may be revealed before you receive the patients' consent to use their data. You have to take care that the documentation of such data does not compromise privacy (for example, it should be strictly anonymous).

Forms for documentation should support the selection process with the inclusion and exclusion criteria clearly laid out. Each single criterion has to be marked whether it is met or not. If any one criterion is not met it usually means that the patient is not eligible and the process is stopped. If possible, pilot the selection process and its documentation in a few patients before starting the study.

4.7.3 Case studies

Case study 1: Uncontrolled observational study (pilot study)

Case study 1 is a descriptive, observational study without control group evaluating a treatment with special acupuncture needles that are left in situ for 7 days, an uncommon procedure but one frequently used by a particular acupuncturist.

Step 1: Develop inclusion and exclusion criteria & step 2: Assess access to patients

In this study steps 1 and 2 are closely linked. Andrew (the investigator) is already using this technique in his own patients regularly. We would thus suggest that he checks his files for patients who have previously received this therapy. His selection criteria should match his patients. However, if the study population is too heterogeneous, readers may find it difficult to interpret the study. After some consideration, Andrew decides to choose the following basic inclusion criteria: aged 18 years and over; clinical diagnosis of non-specific chronic low back pain with duration > 3 months and with pain averaging at least 40 mm on a visual analoque scale; written informed consent. He does not predefine any exclusion criteria. Note that, in order to reduce the likelihood of regression to the mean, patients have to have experienced *an average* of 40 mm on the pain intensity VAS during the last three months whereas in the controlled case study 2 the pain intensity refers only to the last 7 days.

Step 3: Plan the screening and inclusion process

The future readers of the study will have to be convinced that the patients included by Andrew are not just those who were most likely to respond. He should carefully document his screening process and make sure that he keeps any arbitrary selection to a minimum.

Case study 2: Randomized double-blind placebo-controlled study

Case study 2 is an efficacy study which is performed within the relevant regulatory framework. The objective of this randomized controlled trial is to evaluate whether two months treatment with Devil's claw is more effective than placebo in patients with chronic low back pain.

Step 1: Develop inclusion and exclusion criteria

To ensure that this efficacy trial includes a well-defined and homogeneous population of patients, strict selection criteria will be applied. Inclusion criteria: aged 40 to 75 years; clinical diagnosis of chronic low back pain; disease duration > 6 months; average pain intensity of 40 mm or more on a 100-mm VAS during the last seven days; use of oral non-steroidal anti-inflammatory drugs only for treating pain in the four weeks prior to treatment. Exclusion criteria: protrusion or prolapse of 1 or more intervertebral discs with concurrent neurological symptoms; radicular pain; prior vertebral column surgery; infectious spondylopathy; low back pain caused by inflammatory, malignant, or autoimmune disease; congenital deformity of the spine (except for slight lordosis or scoliosis); compression fracture caused by osteoporosis; spinal stenosis; spondylolysis or spondylolisthesis.

Step 2: Assess access to patients

The trial is to be performed in five university outpatient pain clinics in which a large number of low back pain patients are seen regularly. However, many of these patients seen in such centers are complicated cases and may thus not be eligible for inclusion. It is therefore sensible to advertise the study elsewhere to increase access to potentially eligible patients.

Step 3: Plan the screening and inclusion process

The number of patients responding to adverts and seen for eligibility checks in routine practice should be documented. It is likely that the majoritiy of these people will not be included and reasons for non-inclusion should be documented. Simple checklists have to be developed for this prescreening. Detailed documentation with inclusion and exclusion criteria needs to be prepared for those patients who are invited and show up for a formal check. Take care that you meet the requirements of informed consent and data safety if you keep data from patients who do not enter the final study phase.

Case study 3: Pragmatic randomized study comparing three groups

Case study 3 is a comparative effectiveness study in a usual care setting. The objective of this pragmatic randomized three-armed trial is to evaluate whether additional acupuncture treatment or yoga is more effective than usual care alone in the treatment of patients with chronic low back pain and whether one these treatments is more effective than the other.

Step 1: Develop inclusion and exclusion criteria

Because this pragmatic study aims to produce results with high external validity the participants should represent those patients for whom the study treatment options would be considered in routine practice. Therefore, the selection criteria should not be too narrow. Inclusion criteria: aged 18 years and over; clinical diagnosis of chronic low back pain with a duration of > 6 months. May have the following diagnoses/symptoms: protrusion or prolapse of one or more intervertebral discs with concurrent neurologic symptoms; prior vertebral column surgery; infectious spondylopathy; low back pain caused by inflammatory, malignant, or autoimmune disease; compression fracture caused by osteoporosis.

Step 2: Assess access to patients

For this trial a large number of patients (n = 600) will have to be recruited. Patients will be recruited in general practices where also usual care is provided. Patients in the intervention groups will in addition be referred to local acupuncture practices or yoga centres. This is a challenging process. Therefore, a careful planning phase is necessary. The investigators start with 30 general practices each of which should recruit about 20 patients from their practice populations. As this is an ambitious target the investigators already have a plan B. As a first step they would advertise the study in the local media and if this is still insufficient some more general practices will be recruited.

Step 3: Plan the screening and inclusion process

To assess whether the results of such a pragmatic study are generalizable it is particularly important to document the selection process carefully. As so many centres are involved the process should be simple and straightforward. For further details see case study 2.

REFERENCES

Linde K, Streng A, Jürgens S, Hoppe A, Brinkhaus B, Witt C et al. Acupuncture for patients with migraine: a randomized controlled trial. JAMA 2005;293:2,118–2,125.

4.8 Outcome measurement

4.8.1 Theoretical background

Outcome measures are a key element of each study and you have to choose them at the planning stage of your study. Traditional 'hard' outcome measures such as mortality and morbidity are often used in oncology to assess the consequences of treatment in a very concrete, measurable way. Practising clinicians, however, know that the quality of care received is at least as important as the patient's death and survival, or whether or not the disease recurs. Treatment decisions have a very concrete impact on many aspects of the patient's life beyond easily measurable outcomes. It is a common problem that these impacts can be difficult to define and even more difficult to measure. Thus, when you plan your study you have to decide which outcome measures are most suitable. Studies always have more than one outcome measure, and very often 5–10 outcome measures are used assessing different aspects. If you plan a confirmatory study you should also decide which of the outcome measures will serve as primary endpoint and which as secondary endpoints. For many conditions, measurement instruments have previously been designed and validated and it is usually preferable to use such validated tools.

> **!** Always bear in mind that choosing the outcome measures is a key factor in your study. It will influence its acceptability by the research community. Plan enough time to screen the literature and to discuss the options with experts in the field.

What are outcome measures?

In clinical studies we want to detect a change over time which gives us an idea if the intervention makes sense. For this we use outcome measures (or outcome parameters).

Outcomes are defined as the result of health care processes and they are used as tools to measure the change from one point in time (usually before an intervention) to another point in time (usually following an intervention). For clinical studies an outcome measure should be standardized and come with explicit instructions for administration and scoring. Any outcome measure should be reliable, valid, and sensitive to the clinical change that occurs over time.

Reliability is how uniformly the test can be repeated when administered on more than one occasion or by more than one person. **Validity** is the extent to which the test measures what it intends to evaluate, i.e. is it asking the right questions? **Sensi-**

4

tivity to change is the ability of the test to detect true change in patients' status over time. A wide selection of standardized measures is available. They range from 'hard' parameters such as (alive versus dead) to laboratory parameters to 'softer' and often simple and short measures such as the Visual Analogue Scale for pain intensity.

!

The measures you use in your study should be widely accepted for the disease in question, simple to use and acceptable to the patient (e.g. not painful).

Categories of outcome measure

There are different categories of outcome measure and it depends on your research question and the context of your trial which is most suitable. Most outcome measures fit into one of the following three categories:

Objective outcome measures

Objective outcome measures are based on 'objective' criteria such as mortality, laboratory parameters, diagnostic procedures (e.g. X-ray, MRI) or tissue diagnosis. They can be used to decide whether the patient has the disease or a particular stage of disease. After the intervention has been applied the same measures are used to check for improvements. The advantage of objective measures is that they are 'hard facts' and reasonably straightforward. The limitations are that more qualitative, patient-centered aspects are not reflected. However, in drug trials aiming for regulatory approval, objective outcome measures are often demanded.

Subjective outcome measures

In the past two decades the situation of clinical research has become more complex. There is increased awareness of the impact of health care on the quality of human life. Therapeutic interventions are directed as much (and perhaps more) to improving the quality of life as to extending it. Subjective outcome measures had to be defined, and then sound methods developed to produce the tools to measure them. A wide range of outcome measures for different diseases is now available, and some instruments are designed to be used for patient self assessment while others need third person assessment. Pain is a good example where subjective outcome measures are needed. An important group of subjective outcome measures are patient-centered outcomes such as health-related quality of life.

A database of outcome measures of particular importance to CAM can be found here: www.outcomesdatabase.org

Patient-centered outcomes

Patient-centered outcomes have become increasingly relevant in clinical studies and various types exist (e.g. patient preference, patient satisfaction). The outcome most commonly used in clinical studies **is health-related quality of life.** Health-related quality of life describes different domains of health as modified by both disease and treatment processes. Health-related quality of life measures can be grouped into two major categories: generic or disease-specific. **Generic measures** assess the overall impact independent of specific disease type, treatment or patient. **Disease-specific measures** tend to be more sensitive tools, and are designed to capture symptoms that are specific to a given medical condition and measure the direct effects of a condition on an individual's quality of life. There are advantages and disadvantages with each type of measure, and these need to be considered. Although it is often ideal to include components of both a generic and a disease-specific tool, complexity and cumbersome administration can limit the practicality of this approach.

Several generic measures have been developed and validated over time. The 36-item Short Form Health Survey (SF-36) is perhaps the best-known method of assessing health related quality of life. It covers the following six domains of health: physical/emotional/social functioning, pain, vitality, and overall well being (Ware & Sherbourne, 1992). In addition, a shorter version of the SF-36, the SF-12, has been developed and validated (Ware et al., 1996).

The EORTC QLQ-C30 (Aaronson et al., 1993) is perhaps the most common instrument used in the oncologic literature to measure health-related quality of life in cancer patients. The EORTC has begun to expand its research to develop more disease-specific tools (e.g., QLQ-PAN26 for pancreatic cancer) which can be used as an adjunct to the generic instrument.

Pain measures

The measurement of pain can be very simple, for example with Visual Analogue Scales for pain intensity, or integrated in more complex instruments such as the neck pain and disability questionnaire. It depends on the disease and type of pain which measurement fits best. Please have a look at the following examples of simple pain scales.

Visual Analogue Scale (VAS)

The VAS (Huskisson, 1974) is widely used to measure subjective pain (➢ Fig. 4.6). On a 100 mm line the patient marks the intensity of pain experienced. One end corresponds to „no pain", the other to "maximum pain imaginable". The distance from the no-pain end to the patient's mark has to be measured and represents the result in mm, and higher values represent more pain.

Numerical Rating Scale (NRS)

With a NRS (Huskisson 1974) the patient can indicate the pain intensity using numbers from 0 to 10; 0 stands for „no pain" and 10 for „maximum pain imaginable" (➢ Fig. 4.7). In the Box-NRS version of the NRS the numbers are printed in small boxes. The patient is expected to mark his/her rating by making a cross on the appropriate number.

Functional Rating Index (FRI) Pain Intensity Subscale

The FRI was developed for spinal pain and includes scales for nine different aspects of life. The scale for pain intensity offers numbers from 0 to 4, corresponding to „no pain", „mild pain", „moderate pain", „intense pain", and „most severe pain" (Feise & Menke, 2001). The patient has to choose the most suitable answer for each item.

Surrogate measures

A surrogate measure (or marker) is a measure (e.g. cholesterol testing) that may correlate with a real endpoint (e.g. heart disease), but does not necessarily have a linear or consistent relationship. It is often also called **biomarker**.

Surrogate measures are used when the primary endpoint occurs rather late (e.g. death), or when the number of expected events is very small, thus making it impractical to conduct a clinical trial to get a relevant number of events.

Safety measures

Safety of treatments plays an important role in medicine and measuring safety is one aim of clinical studies. In most studies safety measures are secondary outcome parameters. Typical safety measures are the number of patients with Adverse Events and Serious Adverse Events.

Adverse events (AE) are all unwanted or undesirable subjective or objective symptoms, disorders, illnesses, diseases or accidents occurring during the study period, no matter whether they are causally related to the study intervention or not. The intensity of AE and SAE and the causal relationship with the study interventions have to be assessed and documented.

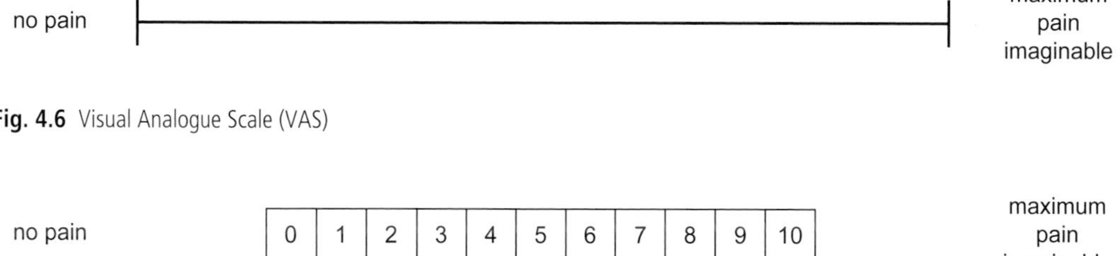

Fig. 4.6 Visual Analogue Scale (VAS)

Fig. 4.7 Numerical Rating Scale (NRS)

4

Adverse effects are all unwanted or undesirable subjective or objective symptoms, disorders, illnesses, diseases or accidents that occur during the study period and are causally related, or possibly causally related, to the study interventions (in the view of the patients or of the study physician).

Serious adverse events (SAE) are all adverse events occurring during the study period which are life-threatening or result in serious harm to health (associated with relevant or permanent disability, necessitating in-patient treatment, involving malignant diseases, medically relevant and leading to a medical intervention to avoid one of the abovementioned problems). For example an accident which leads to a medical intervention is a SAE, even if it is not connected with the study treatment.

SAEs have to be followed up until a final outcome is clear, even if this extends beyond the study period.

There are standards for the terminology used for safety (for more information www.ICH-GCP.org) and it would be helpful to use CRFs from previous studies which have already taken these standards into account.

Further items

Besides outcome measures which aim to measure a change over time, you should document other information about your patients, such as socio demographic data and medical history.

!

Outcome measures and all other aspects which you document together build the case report form (CRF). At the end of your study you have one CRF per patient which includes all data for the particular patient. Depending on the people who provide the information the CRF can have different parts (e.g. patient CRF and practitioner CRF).

When you develop the questions you can use open-ended or closed-ended-questions. **Open-ended questions** are particularly useful when it is important to read what the respondents have to say in their own words. For example: 'What do you think Qigong can do to improve your quality of life?' Open-ended questions leave the respondent free to answer without being limited in any way by the researcher. The disadvantage is that the answers cannot be analyzed with statistical software unless they have been categorized. Another option is to use qualitative research methodology.

Closed-ended questions are more common in clinical research. Typical information in clinical studies includes **socio-demographic data** and medical history. For this you have to develop special items. An **item** consists of a question and options for responses. The method for your response options is dictated, at least in part, by the nature of questions you ask. 'What is your gender?' leads fairly directly to a response method consisting of two boxes one labeled 'female' and the other 'male'. By contrast, the question 'Why did you seek an acupuncturist?' does not dictate a simple two-category response and may require more categories.

In developing response scales, it is helpful to consider the kinds of possible responses which may arise. A basic division is between those responses which are categorical, such as race or staging of breast cancer, and those which are continuous, such as blood pressure (see also categorical and continuous variables in the chapter on basic statistics). A categorical response does not fit into a continuous format, whereas a continuous response can always be categorized.

!

With a continuous variable you develop a continuous response scale which gives you two options for your data analysis. One of them is to calculate continuous measures (e.g. mean and median) and the other is to build categories and to calculate categorical measures (e.g. percentages).

Examples for categorical and continuous responses are shown in ➢ figure 4.8.

Question 4 combines five binary questions and, if you want to ensure that the person who completes the questionnaire reads all of them, you have to use the yes/no response option for each symptom.

Question 5 is an example where only one response can be chosen. In this case use numbers in front of each option to allow valid and fast data entry. For more details ➢ Ch. 5.

Continuous variables

1. How old are you?
   Please fill in your age in years. □□

2. How severe was your average pain in the last 7 days?
   Please mark your average pain intensity on the 100 mm line.
   No pain ├──────────────┤ maximum pain imaginable

Categorical variables

3. Have you ever had an operation on your spine?
   yes □ no □

4. Which of the following symptoms are you currently experiencing?
   a) Headaches yes □ no □
   b) Dizziness yes □ no □
   c) Cough yes □ no □
   d) Sore throat yes □ no □
   e) Back pain yes □ no □
   f) Other: ____________

5. Osteopathy is effective for pain treatment
   a) Strongly agree □
   b) Agree □
   c) Mildly agree □
   d) Disagree □
   e) Strongly disagree □
   f) Don't know □

Fig. 4.8 Examples for categorical and continuous responses

4.8.2 Define your outcome measures and prepare your CRF

Depending on the disease, the research question and the context of your study, choosing the right outcome measures can take a little or a lot of time. Make sure that you allocate enough planning time and get advice from experts in the field.

The most important steps for preparing the outcome measures are:

Define your outcome measures and prepare your measurement instruments	
Step 1	Clarify what you would like to measure
Step 2	Search for existing measurement instruments
Step 3	Develop your own questions
Step 4	Prepare the CRF

Step 1: Clarify what you would like to measure

The first step is to clarify which outcomes you would like to measure. This is also central to your study question (remember the PICO scheme). The outcome measures depend on the disease, the study question and the context of your study. Screen the literature for previous trials for the disease in question and identify the most commonly used measures (e.g. intensity of pain, or back function). Then reflect these measures based onto your study question and context, and decide which of them would be most appropriate as outcomes for your trial. For example, if you plan an efficacy study to bring a new therapy on the market you will need *objective* outcome measures to convince the regulatory bodies. If your focus is more on effectiveness and you plan to provide data for decision making in usual care, then patient centered outcomes should be given preference. If your study is designed as a confirmatory study you have to decide which of your outcomes will be the primary outcome. Give this decision careful consideration, because the interpretation of your study will be mainly based on this parameter. It is common to use disease specific outcome measures as the primary outcome, however, and many studies use health-related quality measures as secondary outcome.

Step 2: Search for existing measurement instruments

After you have identified the outcomes you want to measure, you should perform a literature search screening for existing measurement instruments and also search existing databases (e.g. www.outcomesdatabase.org). In addition, disease specific clinical research or treatment guidelines (e.g. criteria for headache from the International Headache Society) could be very helpful in identifying commonly accepted outcome measures. Having located one or more measures of potential interest you will need to decide which of these is suitable for your study. In part your decision can be guided by a judgment of the appropriateness of the items used in the measurement instrument and the lengths and feasibility of the measurement instrument overall. But the decision should always be supplemented by a critical review of the evidence supporting the instrument. Check if there is convincing evidence on reliability, validity and sensitivity to change for the measurement instruments. Also ask colleagues who have experience with this measurement instrument.

It is preferable to use a previously validated and internationally accepted measurement instrument, but it will also need to be available in your language. For internationally well known validated outcome measurement instruments (e.g. SF-36) you will find validated translations into the most common languages, whereas for other measurement instruments this is not the case.

!

Bear in mind that if you use a validated measurement instrument, it should be available in your language and you have to use it exactly in the format in which it was validated. This includes the order of the items, the types of answers and even the layout. You also need to check if you have to pay for using the measurement instrument.

Step 3: Develop your own questions

After you have decided on the available outcome measures, you may have to develop further items. These items can be descriptive (e.g. age and gender) or serve as further outcomes (e.g. days with pain medication). Be aware that the responses have to correspond with the data (categorical or continuous) and the questions should be clearly phrased.

You always need to collect socio-demographic information. Age, gender and school education are the minimal requirements. Especially in non-randomized studies it would be helpful to have additional information (e.g. current job, family situation, income). Check if there are standard questions for your country. If not, you can use questions which have been used in previous studies.

More complicated is the development of questions to document medical history and inclusion and exclusion criteria. Here you should take into account the common standards for the disease in your study. Screen the literature and seek advice from experts in the field.

If you also want to document medication you should think about the way you will analyze this information. For example if you need the specific days on which pain medication was taken, you have to use a diary. If you want to calculate the average daily dose of a drug you will also need detailed information about the amount of each drug taken by the patient. The documentation of medication is one of the most challenging aspects in clinical studies and you should try to get information from previous studies and discuss your ideas with experts.

You might also be interested in developing questions to assess blinding or patients' expectations. Here again you will find examples in the literature (➤ Ch. 4.6).

Once you have developed your questions you should test them for comprehension and feasibility. Find 5–10 volunteers, ask them to complete the questions and discuss the questionnaire with each person. You can then revise your questions according to the comments.

Step 4: Prepare the case report form

Once you decided on your outcome measures and developed all additional questions (e.g. socio-demographic information and information about the medical history) you have to develop your CRF.

!

The CRF should include only those items which are really necessary. Keep in mind the length of your CRF has an influence on the patients' and practitioners' willingness to complete it.

You have to divide the questions according to who is answering them. If the patient is enrolled by their physician, it may be preferable that the information about the medical history is included in the physicians' case report form (CRF), whereas for example socio-demographic information may be better completed directly by the patient (patient CRF).

!

Be aware that patients who answer questions in front of their physicians could be influenced and this might change the results of your study. If your outcome measure is self assessed by the patient you should ensure that the patient assessment is independent (e.g. by mailing the questionnaire to the patient's home).

You also have to decide which questions from the baseline CRF you want to ask during the follow-up period and whether there will be additional questions only necessary during follow-up (e.g. patient satisfaction or safety information) or only at one follow-up time point (e.g. questions on blinding).

After you have fixed the content of your CRF, you have to decide whether you want to use a paper or an electronic version of your questionnaires. Relevant aspects to be considered for this decision are the size of the study, availability of computers, knowledge of, or support for, developing electronic CRFs and the age of your patients. If you plan a small study and you have only a small budget, then paper questionnaires are still the easiest and safest way of data collection.

4.8.3 Case studies on outcomes

Case study 1: Uncontrolled observational study (pilot study)

Case study 1 is a descriptive, observational study without control group evaluating a treatment with special acupuncture needles left in situ for 7 days, an uncommon procedure but one frequently used by one particular acupuncturist.

Step 1: Clarify what you would like to measure

The main outcome measure should evaluate the intensity of low back pain. Further measures should include other aspects such as quality of life or back function.

Step 2: Search for existing measurement instruments

A literature search for low back pain reveals a number of outcome measures including different pain scales and questionnaires on back function and quality of life. After discussing these with low back pain research experts the following outcome measures are included in the study: low back pain intensity measured on a VAS (0–100mm), back function (HFAQ) and quality of life (SF-36).

Step 3: Develop your own questions

Besides these validated scales, further evaluation items were included such as (1) socio-demographic data: age (continuous variable: years), gender (categorical variable: female/male), school education (categorical variable); (2) medical history: duration of disease (continuous variable: months), medication (drug, dosage), previous diagnostic procedures, previous treatments (categorical variable) and (3) variables such as satisfaction with treatment (categorical variable: very high, high, moderate, low, very low).

Step 4: Prepare your CRF

This is a single center study and the CRF consists of a simple questionnaire for the patients and documentation forms for the practitioner.

4

Case study 2: Randomized double-blind placebo-controlled study

Case study 2 is an efficacy study. The objective of this randomized controlled trial is to evaluate whether a herbal medicine product containing an extract of Harpagophytum procumbens (Devil's claw) and given for two months is more effective than placebo in patients with chronic low back pain.

Step 1: Clarify what you would like to measure

The main outcome measure should evaluate low back pain. Further measures should include further aspects such as quality of life, back function and safety.

Step 2: Search for existing measurement instruments

A literature search for low back pain reveals a number of outcome measures including different pain scales and questionnaires on back function and quality of life. After discussing those with low back pain research experts and screening the most recent international low back pain studies, the 100 mm VAS which measures the average low back pain intensity in the last 7 days is defined as primary outcome. Secondary outcome measures are back function (HFAQ), quality of life (SF-36) and safety (AE and SAE).

Step 3: Develop your own questions

Further questions on socio-demographic characteristics, medical history, other interventions, expectation and blinding are developed.

Step 4: Prepare your CRF

This study is a multi-center study and separate case report forms are developed for patients and physicians. The CRF for each patient is organized according to the study procedures. In addition guidance for the study investigator is provided with notes and flow charts.

Case study 3: Pragmatic randomized study comparing three groups

Case study 3 is a comparative effectiveness study in a usual care setting. The objective of this pragmatic randomized three-armed trial is to evaluate whether additional acupuncture treatment or yoga is more effective than usual care alone in the treatment of patients with chronic low back pain and whether one of these treatments is more effective than the other.

Step 1: Clarify what you would like to measure

In this pragmatic study, a measure which reflects back function is defined as the primary outcome. In addition quality of life should be measured.

Step 2: Search for existing measurement instruments

A literature search for low back pain reveals a number of outcome measures for back function and quality of life. After discussing those with low back pain research experts and screening the most recent low back pain studies from Germany, the HFAQ questionnaire on back function is defined as the primary outcome measure and the SF-36 (quality of life) and safety (SAE) as secondary outcome measures. Although the HFAQ is mainly used in Germany it is used in this study, because the study gathers data for decision making in Germany.

Step 3: Develop your own questions

Further questions on socio-demographic characteristics, medical history, further interventions and expectation are developed.

Step 4: Prepare your CRF

The CRF for patients and the study centres is web based.

REFERENCES

Aaronson NK, Ahmedzai S, Bergman B, Bullinger M, Cull A, Duez NJ et al. The European Organization for Research and Treatment of Cancer QLQ-C30: a quality-of-life instrument for use in international clinical trials in oncology. J Natl Cancer Inst 1993;85:365–76.

Feise R., Menke M. (2001). Functional Rating Index: A New Valid and Reliable Instrument to Measure the Magnitude of Clinical Change in Spinal Conditions. Spine, 26(1), 78–87.

Huskisson E.C. 1974. Measurement of Pain. The Lancet, 9, 1,127–1,131.

Ware JE, Kosiknski M, Keller SD. A 12-item short form health survey: construction of scales and preliminary tests of reliability and validity. Med Care 1996;34(3).

Ware JE, Sherbourne CD. The MOS 36-item short-form health survey (SF-36). I. Conceptual framework and item selection. Med Care 1992;30(6):473–83. 220–3.

4.9 Sample size calculation

This chapter aims to give basic insights into sample size calculation and how the assumptions of clinicians influence this.

4.9.1 What does sample size calculation mean?

If you throw a coin ten times and you get "head" seven times and "tails" three times, you would not necessarily think that there is something wrong with the coin. This result could well be due to chance. But if you throw it a hundred times and you still get "tails" in only 30 % you would be quite sure that this is no longer due to chance. There must be something seriously wrong with that coin! With 100 throws you have quite high sensitivity to detect a serious deviation from what you would expect from throwing an unbiased coin. However, imagine you throw another coin 100 times and you come up with "tails" 40 times. This is less than you might expect but it might simply be chance. But if you throw it a thousand times and it still comes up with tails only 40 % of the time, this is quite suspicious.

In clinical trials it is crucial to be able to tell chance from a true effect. It is obvious that you will not need very many patients if you have a big difference in outcomes between two treatments. If, however, the difference is small then you need many more patients to detect it with reasonable certainty. Patients are individuals who do not react in a very predictable manner to treatment and measurement errors occur. Sample size calculation helps you to determine how many patients should be included in your study.

!

> The definitive sample size calculation of your trial should be performed by a statistician. But the most important assumptions for the sample size calculation come from the clinician/researcher and small changes in the assumptions can dramatically change the sample sizes calculated. Therefore, clinicians should have a basic idea of the principles of sample size calculation.
> As this chapter does not aim to give a comprehensive introduction into sample size calculation, we will only discuss the most frequent and straightforward case: two-armed randomized trial testing whether the outcomes in the two groups differ. But obviously, sample size calculations can be done for many other studies (e.g. Katz 2006).

Basic sample size calculations for two-armed trials are simple and can be performed without a computer. For the novice or clinician this is a great chance to see that there is nothing magic about it and to get a sense of how assumptions influence the number of patients needed. Nevertheless, in planning an actual clinical study appropriate software programs should be used.

A number of free software tools for sample size calculations are available from the internet. Here are three examples:

- EpiCalc is a Windows application and can be downloaded at www.brixtonhealth.com/epicalc.

4

html. It is a simple general statistical calculator for pre-tabulated data which includes a basic function for sample size calculation. We would not recommend using EpiCalc for the final sample size calculation, but for running preliminary calculations it is easy to use even for researchers with only basic knowledge. Therefore, we use this program for the calculations in the different steps described below.
- Simple Interactive Statistical Analysis (SISA) at www.quantitativeskills.com/sisa/calculations/samsize.htm is an online tool for two-group comparisons.
- G*Power can be downloaded at www.psycho.uni-duesseldorf.de/abteilungen/aap/gpower3/ and is a slightly more advanced and professional Windows tool. We use G*Power for calculating sample sizes for the case studies.

Biostatisticians either use power calculation functions built into major statistical programs such as STATA, or specialized commercial software such as NQuery Advisor or PASS. An overview of sample size software can be found on a website of the Department of Epidemiology & Biostatistics at the University of California, San Francisco (www.epibiostat.ucsf.edu/biostat/sampsize.html).

4.9.2 Practical steps

Steps of a sample size calculation	
Step 1	Decide on the outcome measure for calculations
Step 2	Define what you are looking for
Step 3	Decide on the significance level, the power and whether you will test one- or two-sided
Step 4	Decide on a clinically meaningful difference and run preliminary calculations
Step 5	Check how sensitive the calculations react to your assumptions
Step 6	What can you do if the calculated sample size is too large?

Step 1: Decide on the outcome measure for calculations

Before starting to do any number crunching you have to decide the outcome measure you will base your calculations on. Normally this should be your main outcome measure. For example, in a depression trial this may be a particular patient response (e.g. a clinically relevant improvement). This is – remember ➤ chapter 3 – a dichotomous outcome (the response can only be 'yes' or 'no'). In a trial on pain, the main outcome could be the post-treatment value on a 100 mm VAS (so the result can be any value between 0 and 100) – thus a continuous measure. In some situations it can be more difficult to choose the outcome for the sample size calculation, for example if you have both symptom severity and rescue medication use (which influence each other) as main outcomes. In such cases one outcome measure is usually selected; criteria for selection are typically clinical relevance, whether the outcome can be measured reliably in the trial, and whether information facilitating sample size calculations (data from previous studies) is available. Alternatively, sample size calculations can be done for both outcomes.

Step 2: Define what you are looking for

After deciding on the outcome measure you have to clarify what you are investigating: whether your treatment intervention is superior to the control, whether it is equivalent or whether it is non-inferior. These concepts have been introduced in ➤ chapter 3. If your trial has more than two groups, or if you go for equivalence or non-inferiority, or if you have a randomized trial with complex multivariate analyses or cluster randomization you will need to involve a statistician straightaway; there is no point in having a go at any calculations yourself.

Step 3: Decide on the significance level, the power and whether your test will be one- or two-sided

This step is probably the most difficult one for clinicians to understand as it involves several inter-related statistical concepts. You need to fix the significance level, the power and whether your test will be one- or two sided. The background for this is hypothesis testing which has been explained in ➢ chapter 3 and which is briefly repeated here.

Imagine two studies investigating whether a Hypericum extract is better than placebo for treating depression. Study 1 uses 1 mg extract per day – a dose where we do not expect any effect at all, while study 2 uses 900 mg – a dose which is expected to be effective.

As you (hopefully) remember from ➢ chapter 3 a statistical hypothesis always consists of a **null hypothesis** (H_0) which usually assumes no effect (e.g. there is no difference between the Hypericum and placebo) and an **alternative hypothesis** (H_A) which holds the null hypothesis not to be true (e.g. Hypericum is different from placebo).

In our study 1 using a clearly sub-therapeutic dose of Hypericum extract, we can be quite certain that H_0 is true. If study 1 does not find a difference between Hypericum and placebo H_0 stays and this would be correct (see cell 1 in ➢ table 4.4). However, it is possible that, although Hypericum in that dosage is not effective, we may still find a difference just by chance. In that case we would reject H_0 although it is true (cell 3 in ➢ table 4.4). Our study would be **false positive** and we would commit a so-called type α- **(alpha) error**. For each study we have to fix what likelihood of an α-error is acceptable and so at what point we consider a result as significant. The most common value for an acceptable type α-error is 0.05 or 5 %. This is also called **significance level** of 0.05 or 5 %. Once you have your data, after conducting the study, you can calculate the p-value which estimates the probability that you commit an α-error. If the p-value is below 0.05 you reject the H_0 as it is below your predefined level, but if it is 0.05 or above you accept it.

Consider now Study 2. Here the "truth" should be that 900 mg Hypericum extract is indeed more effective than a placebo. If you find such a difference in your study (with a p-value below 0.05) you correctly reject H_0 (cell 4 in ➢ table 4.4). However, it may happen that the p-value in your study is above 0.05 and you erroneously accept H_0. In this case our study is **false negative** and we commit a so-called type β-**(beta) error** (cell 2 in ➢ table 4.4). Typical values for an acceptable type β-error are 0.2 (20 %) or 0.1 (10 %).

You may have heard that sample size calculation is sometimes also called power calculation. Statistical **power** is the likelihood that you will reject the null hypothesis when the effects of your treatment indeed differ from those of the control treatment to the extent that you assume. Power is calculated by subtracting the β-error from 1 (1–β). So if you accept a β-error of 0.2 (or 20 %) the power of your trial is 80 %, and if you only accept a β-error of 0.1 (or 10 %) the power is 90 %. You can probably imagine that to achieve greater power you need more patients.

For the sample size calculation you have to fix the significance level (or an acceptable α-error) and the power (or an acceptable β-error). But this is still not enough.

You also have to decide whether calculations will be run for a one-sided (only looking whether your Hypericum is *superior* to placebo) or a two-sided (looking whether Hypericum is *superior or inferior* to placebo) hypothesis test. This is explained in detail in chapter 3. Unless you have very good reasons to use a one-sided test choose a two-sided test to be on the safe side.

If your randomization ratio differs from 1 : 1 you have to account for it in the calculation. The total number of participants needed is lowest for a ratio of 1 : 1.

Table 4.4 Errors in hypothesis-testing

	Truth	
Decision	H0 is true	H0 not true
Accept H0	✓ Cell 1	β-error Cell 2
Reject H0	Cell 3 α-error (significance level)	Cell 4 ✓ (power)

Step 4: Decide on a clinically meaningful difference and run preliminary calculations

!

Step 4 is the most crucial in the process, and one for which clinical knowledge is much more important than statistical knowledge. So do not hand over the responsibility for this step to the statistician!
Step 4 depends on whether the main outcome measure used for the sample size calculation is continuous or dichotomous.

4

Testing whether a continuous outcome differs between two groups

If your outcome is continuous you have to fix two values: 1) the minimum clinically relevant difference between the means in the two groups, and 2) the expected standard deviations for these two means. Whenever possible you should get information on these values from the literature and/or a pilot study. When using data from the literature look on the findings of large and rigorous studies and do not rely on the assumptions of sample size calculations in small studies as these are often overoptimistic.

!

By dividing the expected difference between the two means in the two groups by the assumed standard deviation you calculate the standardized difference (syn. standardized mean difference, Cohen's d, sometimes also simply called effect size).
For example, quite a number of pain trials have used optimistic assumptions like this: they expected that, after the intervention, patients in the treatment group would report a mean pain intensity of 20 on the 100 mm VAS compared to 50 in the control group. The standard deviations of the means were estimated to be 30 mm in both groups. If you divide the difference between the two means (30 mm in our example) by the standard deviation (also 30 mm in our example) the resulting standardized difference is 1. As you will see below, the standardized difference has a key role for sample size calculation.

With the difference between the means of the two groups, the standard deviation (or the standardized difference calculated from these two) and the values decided on in step 3 (significance level, for power – or beta-, one- or two-sided test). Your statistician can now run the calculation (see the following table 4.5). However, to get a feeling of what's going you can do some estimations or calculations easily yourself. You can use some of the software indicated in the first part of this chapter, but we do it here without a computer. Altman's nomogram (➤ Fig. 4.9) is a very simple graphical tool to crudely estimate the sample size needed in a two-group comparison. On the left you have a scale with standardized differences, on the right you have a scale where you can choose the power level, in between you have the total number of patients needed for two widely used significance levels (0.05 and 0.01).

Table 4.5 Summary of parameters to fix when performing a sample size calculation for a two-group comparison with a continuous outcome

Parameter	Value
Allocation ratio: treatment to control	usually 1 : 1
Significance level (alpha)	most often 5 % (sometimes 1 %)
Power	often 80 % (quite often higher)
Test	usually two-sided
Difference between means in experimental and control group*	if possible based on literature review, pilot study; and/or clinical reasoning
Standard deviation in experimental and control group*	if possible based on literature review, pilot study and/or clinical reasoning

* You can also give your statistician the standardized difference which is calculated by dividing the difference between the two means by the standard deviation

Based on the assumptions for our pain study, we have calculated a standardized difference of 1. If you draw a line between the standardized difference of 1 and the usual power level of 80 % you find on the scale in the middle that you will need about 32 (2 × 16) patients if your significance level is 5 % and about 46 (2 × 23) patients if you choose a significance level of 1 %. For a power of 90 % and a significance level of 5 % you need 40 (2 × 23) patients, for a significance level of 1 % 60 (2 × 30) patients. Entering the appropriate values into one (G*Power version 3.1.2) of the cited free available software tools yielded very similar values (➤ Fig. 4.9).

Testing whether a dichotomous outcome differs between two groups

If your outcome is binary the only thing you need to fix is the frequency of events in the two groups. For example, if you plan to do a placebo-controlled trial of a Hypericum extract for depression you can look at the response rates previously reported in placebo groups of antidepressant trials. Often these are around 30 %. You should then define the minimal clinically relevant difference. Sometimes you will

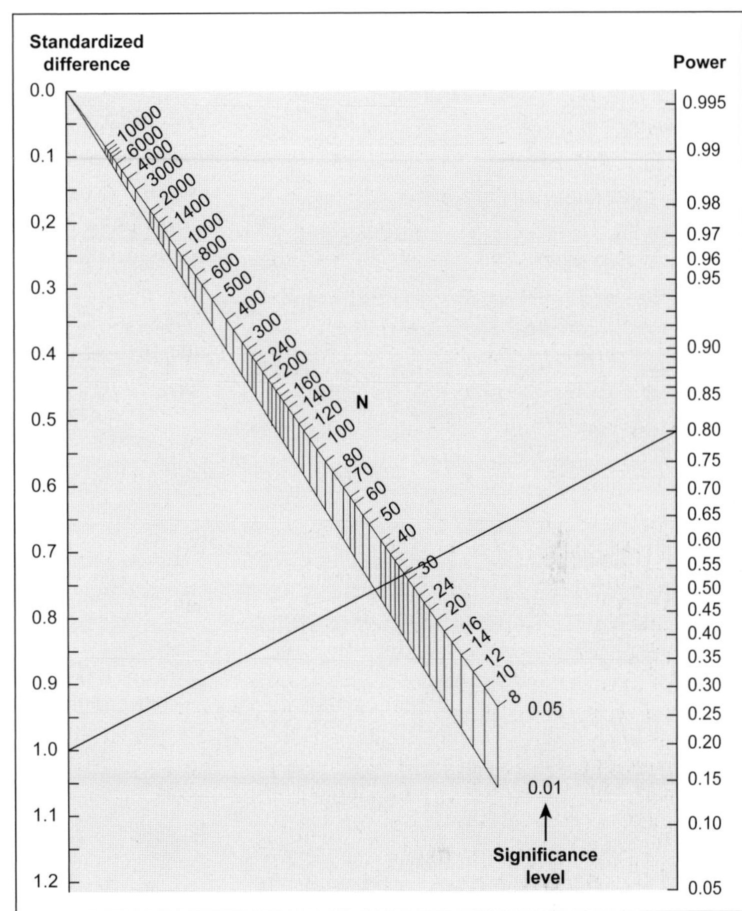

Fig. 4.9 Altman's nomogram – sample size needed for a trial with a standardized difference of 1.0 and 80 % power. Modified from Altman (1982) by courtesy of Blackwell Publishing

find guidelines for such differences in the literature or you will find typical assumptions in clinical trials. For example, you could say that at least 50 % of patients receiving the new treatment (20 % more than with placebo) should be responders. These assumptions together with the issues fixed at step 3 are all you need to run the calculations (see the following table). If you use the typical parameter values of 5 % for the significance level (α), 80 % for power and a two-sided hypothesis test a sample size calculation using one of the programs listed above (G*Power 3.1.2) reveals that you will need 102 patients in each group (a total of 204 patients) (➤ Table 4.6):

Table 4.6 Summary of parameters that need to be fixed when performing a sample size calculation for a two-group comparison for a dichotomous outcome

Allocation ratio: treatment to control	usually 1 : 1
Significance level (alpha)	most often 5 % (sometimes 1 %)
Power	often 80 % (quite often higher)
Test	almost always two-sided
Control group event rate	if possible based on literature review or pilot study
Minimal important difference/Test group event rate	if possible based on literature review and clinical reasoning

4

You can also use Altman's nomogram for dichotomous outcomes, but you need to do some algebra first for calculating the standardized difference (see the following box).

How to calculate the standardized difference from two proportions

$$\text{Standardized difference} = \frac{Pe - Pc}{P(1-P)}$$

P_e = Proportion of events in the experimental group
P_c = Proportion of events in the control group

$$P = \frac{Pe + Pc}{2}$$

Applied to our example of the Chinese herbs for depression with $P_e = 0.5$ and $P_c = 0.3$

$$P = \frac{0.5 + 0.3}{2} = \frac{0.8}{2} = 0.4$$

Standardized difference

$$= \frac{0.5 - 0.3}{0.4\,(1-0.4)} = \frac{0.2}{0.4\,(0.6)} = \frac{0.2}{0.24} = \frac{0.2}{0.49} = 0.41$$

Accounting for drop-outs

It is common practice to add 10 to 20 % more patients to the number estimated by the sample size calculation to account for drop-outs or missing data. This is particularly relevant if missing data will not be replaced in your trial, but many replacement techniques are also associated with some loss of power.

Step 5: Check how sensitive the calculations are to your assumptions

A huge problem with the assumptions for sample size calculations is that they are a) often very uncertain, and b) often overoptimistic. Assuming a standardized difference of 1 for a trial comparing, for example, acupuncture for headache to no treatment is overoptimistic, for a trial comparing acupuncture with sham acupuncture it is simply unrealistic. As a rule of thumb, standardized differences up to 0.39 are considered small effects, from 0.4 to 0.69 moderate effects, and those above 0.7 are large effects. In CAM research, effects versus placebo or sham, if you find any, are often small and sometimes moderate, and effects versus no treatment or waiting list are often moderate and only occasionally large.

Small changes in your assumptions can have dramatic consequences. For example, if we assume that in our pain trial the post treatment pain intensity on the VAS is 30 instead of 20 mm (resulting in a standardized difference of 0.67; ➤ Table 4.7) we then need 74 (2 × 37) patients to achieve 80 % of power with a standard deviation still at 30 mm. If you do a sham-controlled trial it might be prudent to only assume 10 mm difference (standardized difference 0.33) in pain intensity as sham acupuncture interventions are often associated with surprising analgesic effects. In that case you would need 286 (2 × 143) patients (➤ Table 4.7).

Table 4.7 Examples for sample sizes needed for a continuous outcome. Calculations performed with G*Power 3.1.2

					Patients needed (in two groups) under following conditions		
Mean treatment group	Mean control group	Difference between means	Standard deviation	**Standardized difference**	α = 5 % Power = 80 % two-sided test	α = 5 % Power = 90 % two-sided test	α = 1 % Power = 90 % two-sided test
20	50	30	30	**1**	2 × 17	2 × 23	2 × 32
30	50	20	30	**0.67**	2 × 37	2 × 49	2 × 69
35	50	15	30	**0.5**	2 × 64	2 × 86	2 × 121
40	50	10	30	**0.33**	2 × 143	2 × 191	2 × 270
45	50	5	30	**0.17**	2 × 567	2 × 758	2 × 1,073
30	50	30	20	**1**	2 × 17	2 × 23	2 × 32
40	50	10	20	**0.5**	2 × 64	2 × 86	2 × 121

With dichotomous outcomes the situation is, in principle, the same. However, as dichotomous outcomes carry less information than continuous outcomes (for example above or below 50 mm versus any possible value on the 100 mm VAS), trials with binary outcomes in general need larger sample sizes. If you assume for our 'depression' example that the response rate in the placebo control group is 35 % instead of 30 % the number of patients needed increases to 183 per group, and if the response rate in the placebo group is 40 % you need 404 per group! If you think a power of 80 % is insufficient or if you want to use a more rigorous significance level the sample size needed increases further (➤ Table 4.8).

Be aware that it is not only the absolute difference between the two groups which influences the sample size calculation but also the frequency of events. In our table showing examples, the sample size needed to detect a difference of 10 % is 2 × 404 (with $\alpha = 5$ % and a power of 80 % and a two-sided test) if the control group event rate is 40 %, but 2 × 151 if the control group event rate is 15 %.

!

Since your assumptions have such a huge impact on your calculated sample size we recommend that you check the impact of changing these assumptions within realistic limits.

Step 6: What can you do if the calculated sample size is too large?

Unfortunately, when using realistic and careful assumptions, you might often end up with a sample size beyond your recruitment possibilities. It is NOT a good strategy to simply manipulate your assumptions until you get your preferred sample size! So what can you do?

One option is to abandon the trial. It is unethical and an abuse of limited resources to perform studies which do not produce meaningful answers. If only a sufficiently powered trial is acceptable then this may be the only option. However, in the age of meta-analyses carefully performed underpowered trials can be ethical and useful. However, if you are aware that your trial is underpowered you will need good arguments for performing it.

Obviously, you should consider whether there are realistic strategies to successfully recruit the number of patients needed, for example by including further study centers, by prolonging the recruitment period, by eliminating any dispensable inclusion or exclusion criteria etc. However, be careful, as including further centers or changing inclusion criteria might also have an influence on differences between groups or on variability.

If the sample size needed remains unrealistic and you still want to do the trial you could consider whether there is a more sensitive marker of the out-

Table 4.8 Examples for sample sizes needed for a binary outcome (response). Calculations performed with G*Power 3.1.2

		Patients needed (in two groups) under the following conditions		
Responder rate Treatment group	Responder rate Control group	$\alpha = 5$ % Power = 80 % two-sided test	$\alpha = 5$ % Power = 90 % two-sided test	$\alpha = 1$ % Power = 90 % two-sided test
50 %	20 %	2 × 44	2 × 58	2 × 79
50 %	30 %	2 × 102	2 × 133	2 × 186
50 %	35 %	2 × 183	2 × 242	2 × 332
50 %	40 %	2 × 404	2 × 533	2 × 751
50 %	45 %	2 × 1,606	2 × 2,124	2 × 3,001
15 %	5 %	2 × 151	2 × 198	2 × 279
10 %	5 %	2 × 466	2 × 606	2 × 845

4

come. For example, many cardiovascular studies do not focus on one selected outcome such as myocardial infarction but use so-called composite outcomes, such as any major event (including myocardial infarction, stroke, hospitalization, coronary surgery, and percutaneous coronary intervention). The occurrence of at least one of these outcomes is much more likely than of myocardial infarction alone and, thus decreases the number of patients needed to detect a clinically relevant difference. In a number of conditions, summary scores integrating several symptoms influenced by the treatment can increase sensitivity. However, often the variation of summary scores is increased when compared to single symptoms and the real increase in power is thus limited.

Repeated measurement of the outcome in the same subjects also increases power. Sample size calculations and analyses for repeated measurements are more complex but your statistician will be able to deal with that.

If your power is, for example, 90 % or your significance 1 % you can consider relaxing these to the usual thresholds of 80 % and 5 %. Going further is not advisable with only few exceptions. Depending on the specific situations there may be other ways of increasing power; so seek advice from experienced researchers in your area.

4.9.3 Case studies

Case study 1: Uncontrolled observational study (pilot study)

Case study 1 is a descriptive, observational study without control group evaluating a treatment with special acupuncture needles left in situ for 7 days, an uncommon procedure but one frequently used by a particular acupuncturist.

Step 1: Decide on the outcome measure for calculations

As this is an uncontrolled pilot study a sample size calculation is only performed to get a crude idea whether expected changes over time would be significant. Back pain intensity on the VAS is used as outcome measure for calculations.

Step 2: Define what you are looking for

This study looks on differences between VAS values before and after treatment.

Step 3: Decide on the significance level, the power and whether your test will be one- or two-sided

We choose the usual values: significance level (and alpha) 5 %, 80 % power and two-sided testing

Step 4: Decide on a clinically meaningful difference and run preliminary calculations

To be clinically relevant, the difference between before and after treatment should be at least 15 mm assuming a standard deviation of 30 mm. G*Power calculates a sample size needed of 36 patients. Assuming a drop-out rate of 10 % 40 patients are set as recruitment target.

Step 5: Check how sensitive your calculations are to your assumptions

Not done for this pilot study

Step 6: What can you do if the calculated sample size is too large?

The recruitment of 40 patients seems realistic for the study.

Case study 2: Randomized double-blind placebo-controlled study

Case study 2 is an efficacy study. The objective of this randomized controlled trial is to evaluate whether an herbal medicine product containing an extract of Harpagophytum procumbens (Devil's claw) and given for two months is more effective than placebo in patients with chronic low back pain.

Step 1: Decide on the outcome measure for calculations

As discussed in chapter 4.8 the primary outcome is low back pain intensity in the last 7 days measured on a 100 mm VAS (time point for confirmatory analysis 2 months after randomization = end of treatment).

Step 2: Define what you are looking for

On a clinical level this trial investigates whether Devil's claw is superior to placebo (superiority) but in accordance with usual approaches in statistical testing it will investigate whether Devil's claw is *different* from placebo.

Step 3: Decide on the significance level, the power and whether your test will be one- or two-sided

We choose the usual values: significance level (and alpha) 5 %, 80 % power and a two-sided test.

Step 4: Decide on a clinically meaningful difference and run preliminary calculations

A mean difference of 10 mm on the VAS is considered the minimal clinically relevant effect. If a standard deviation of 20 mm is assumed for both groups this would result in a standardized difference of 0.5. According to calculations with the software G*Power, the sample size needed is 64 patients per group (128 in total). To account for a drop-out of about 10 % a recruitment target of 140 patients is considered appropriate.

Step 5: Check how sensitive your calculations are to your assumptions

If the true standard deviation is wider (keeping the mean difference equal to step 4), considerably more patients would be needed to keep 80 % power: with a standard deviation of 25 mm (resulting in a standardized difference of 0.4) 2 × 100 patients would be needed, and with a standard deviation of 30 mm (resulting in a standardized difference of 0.33) 2 × 143 patients.

Step 6: What can you do if the calculated sample size is too large?

With the five centers in the study a recruitment target of 140 patients seems realistic.

Case study 3: Pragmatic randomized study comparing three groups

Case study 3 is a comparative effectiveness study in a usual care setting. The objective of this pragmatic randomized three-armed trial is to evaluate whether additional acupuncture treatment or Yoga is more effective in the treatment of patients with chronic low back pain than usual care alone and whether acupuncture is more effective than Yoga.

Step 1: Decide on the outcome measure for calculations

4

The primary outcome is back function measured by the HFAQ after three months (➤ Ch. 4.8).

Step 2: Define what you are looking for

On a clinical level this trial investigates whether acupuncture or Yoga given alongside usually care is superior to usual care alone (superiority) but in accordance with usual approaches in statistical testing it will investigate whether these treatments are *different* from usual care (they could be harmful). The comparison of acupuncture versus Yoga is a secondary aim for which no sample size calculation is done.

Step 3: Decide on the significance level, the power and whether your test will be one- or two-sided

As two comparisons (acupuncture vs. usual care and Yoga vs. usual care) will be tested a significance level (and alpha) of 2.5 % is chosen instead of 5 %; 80 % power and two-sided testing.

Step 4: Decide on a clinically meaningful difference and run preliminary calculations

A mean difference of 10 mm on the VAS is considered the minimal clinically relevant effect. As inclusion criteria are wide a standard deviation of 30 mm is assumed for both groups. The resulting standardized difference is 0.33. According to calculations with the software G*Power, the sample size needed is 176 patients per group (528 in total). To account for a drop-out of about 15 % a recruitment target of 600 patients is considered appropriate.

Step 5: Check how sensitive your calculations are to your assumptions

The assumptions in this calculation are quite conservative (a standardized difference of 0.33). If it had been 0.4 instead, then 121 patients per group would have been sufficient.

Step 6: What can you do if the calculated sample size is too large?

4

With the infrastructure and funding available the recruitment target of 600 patients is realistic. If recruitment progresses too slowly the inclusion of further study centers would be the first option.

REFERENCES

Katz MH. Study design and statistical analysis. A practical guide for clinicians. Cambridge: Cambridge University Press, 2006.

4.10 Ethics and regulatory aspects

4.10.1 Theoretical background on ethics

We have to consider ethical issues whenever patients or healthy volunteers are included in studies. This chapter summarizes the rationale behind ethical approval and provides practical advice for your study.

Declaration of Helsinki

A set of ethical principles for clinical studies has been developed by the World Medical Association and is called the **Declaration of Helsinki** (www.wma.net/e/policy/b3.htm). Although it is not a legally binding instrument, it is widely regarded as a key document for ethics in clinical research. The fundamental principle is respect for the individual (Article 8), the right to self determination and the right to make informed decisions with regards to participation in research (Articles 20, 21 and 22). While there is always a need for research (Article 6), the subject's welfare must always take precedence over the interests of science and society (Article 5), and ethical considerations must always take precedence over laws and regulations (Article 9).

Institutional Review Board (IRB)/Ethics Committees

Your research should be guided by the Declaration of Helsinki and each clinical study has to have approval from the appropriate **Institutional Review Board (IRB)** in the US or the appropriate **Ethics Committees** in Europe. Their function is to perform a critical review on any research conducted on human subjects with regards to science, ethics, and regulations.

According to ICH GCP guidelines (www.ich.org)

- The IRB/Ethics Committee should safeguard the rights, safety, and well-being of all study participants.
- Special attention should be paid to studies that may include vulnerable subjects, such as pregnant women, children, prisoners, elderly, or persons with impaired comprehension.
- The IRB/Ethics Committee may only approve research
  - for which there is an informed consent process for participants,
  - for which the risks to the subjects are balanced by potential benefits to society, and
  - for which the selection of subjects presents a fair or just distribution of risks and benefits to eligible participants.

IRB/Ethics Committees should involve groups of individuals from diverse backgrounds (healthcare professionals and non-medical members), whose responsibility it is to protect the rights, safety and well-being of human subjects involved in a clinical study. The IRB/Ethics Committee needs the following documents as minimal requirement:

- Study protocol
- Written informed consent form
- Patient information leaflet

- Patient recruitment procedures (e.g. advertisements),
- Investigator's Brochure (IB) for drug trials including available safety information
- Information about payments and compensation available to subjects
- The investigator's current curriculum vitae and/or other documentation providing evidence of qualifications and competence

The IRB/Ethics Committee will continue to review each ongoing study and must be informed about any changes (e.g. study protocol, patient informed consent form, and patient information). Any new information is called 'amendment'.

4.10.2 Getting approval from the IRB/Ethics Committee

Depending on the country and the content of your study, getting approval from the IRB/Ethics Committee can be challenging and time consuming. You should thus prepare an approval application at the beginning of your study.

!

> Keep in mind that you need ethical approval for most studies and that you cannot start your study before it is approved.

The most important steps for successful ethical approval are:

Getting approval from IRB/Ethics Committee	
Step 1	Identify the appropriate IRB/Ethics Committee
Step 2	Check the format for the application
Step 3	Check the time line
Step 4	Be prepared when defending your study

Step 1: Identify the appropriate IRB/Ethics Committee

Before you seek ethical approval you have to identify the IRB/Ethics Committee which is responsible for your study. Double check this as preparing the documents for the wrong one will be time- and work-consuming. If you plan a multi-center study you should clarify the procedure. It depends on the regulations of your country whether you can apply centrally or whether you have to apply in each county separately.

Step 2: Check the format for the application

Having identified the appropriate IRB/Ethics Committee, you should check their requirements in terms of content and format. Most provide detailed information on their websites. It is important that you prepare all the documents needed in the suggested format, because most IRBs/Ethics Committees do a formal check of the application before they start the process and queries can be time-consuming.

The patient information leaflet and the patient informed consent form are key documents. They should be clearly written using a language which is understandable for lay people. Most IRBs/Ethics Committees have checklists or examples for download on their website.

Find out if there are any fees to pay.

Step 3: Check the time line

Getting ethical approval can often be time consuming which must be taken into account when planning the study. If your documents are badly prepared it is likely to cost you extra time but even well prepared documents can take longer than planned. Check the timeline for the IRB/Ethics Committee in advance (dates for sending the application, dates for consultations, time allowed for modifications) and integrate this information into the timeline of your study.

Step 4: Be prepared when defending your study

Most IRB/Ethics Committees invite the principal investigator to be present at the heading, and sometimes to make a presentation. You should make sure you are well prepared to present and defend your study in front of the IRB/Ethics Committee. You should know your documents and study methods in detail and have a copy of each document you have sent to them present at the discussion.

The IRB/Ethics Committee has three options for a decision:

- Approval/favourable opinion
- Modifications required prior to approval/favourable opinion;
- Disapproval/negative opinion

In addition, a termination or suspension of any prior approval or favourable opinion is possible during the trial period.

!

Always keep in mind that the focus of the IRB/Ethics Committee is on safeguarding the rights, safety, and well-being of all study participants. Because of this, patient information, the patient informed consent form and the risk-benefit ratio will be central to the discussion.

4.10.3 Regulatory aspects

Regulatory aspects differ from country to country and depend on the intervention you want to study. For example, in most countries drug trials are much more regulated than non-pharmaceutical studies. In addition to the approval from the IRB/Ethics Committee, a drug trial also needs approval by state institutions responsible for drug and medical devices (e.g. FDA in the US, EMEA in Europe or BfArM in Germany). Standard forms and procedures for application to those institutions are usually available on their respective websites and should be followed to avoid problems. The documentation for drug trials must follow the ICH-GCP guidelines. Preparing the application and managing the trial are both more resource intensive than in non-pharmaceutical trials.

CHAPTER 5 Study and data management

An important part of your study is the management of the study itself and of the data. This chapter will give an overview of the most important aspects of study and data management.

5.1 Project management

Project management plans, organizes and manages processes to allow successful completion of specific project objectives. The primary challenge of project management is to achieve all of these objectives within the limits of the known constraints of the project such as scope, time and budget. A further challenge is to optimize the allocation of resources to meet the objectives as efficiently as possible.

5.1.1 Phases of project management

Most projects have at least five phases (➤ Fig. 5.1).

In a clinical study you have to manage all five phases. The initiation and planning phases are already completed when you start your study. The execution of the trial is a complicated and time consuming phase and is closely connected to the monitoring and controlling of all processes. You will only achieve good quality data and successful completion of your trial if you provide good interaction between execution and monitoring/controlling.

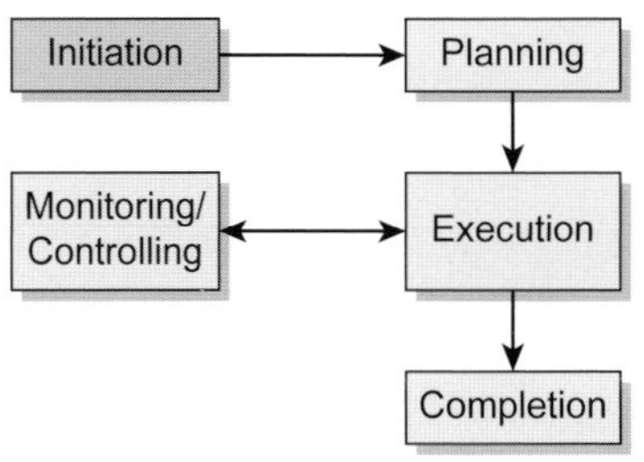

Fig. 5.1 Different phases of project management

There is a large amount of literature about project management theory, tools and software. This is useful if you plan to be a project manager for large scale clinical studies. However, if you only want to run smaller studies you do not need to go deeply into details of project management. In the section 'managing your study' we will summarize the most important aspects of successful study management.

5.1.2 Taking notes

Taking notes in a structured way is helpful when managing your trial. There are two main options: checklists and mind maps.

Checklists

Checklists are the most common way of taking notes. The main facts are just listed and can be sorted according to the time line or their importance.

Mind Mapping

Mind Mapping is a technique which uses a more creative way of taking notes. Instead of listing the aspects of your study you map them in a structured network (➤ Fig. 5.2). The advantage of Mind Maps is that you can quickly identify and understand the structure of a topic, and the way pieces of information fit together. They can be used for summarizing information, consolidating information from different research sources, thinking through complex problems or presenting information in a format that shows the overall structure of your study.

If you want to try Mind Mapping yourself you will find a short introduction in the following box.

!

Write the title of the subject you are exploring in the center of the page, and draw a box (or circle) around it. This is shown in the center marked '1 recruitment' in ➤ figure 5.2.
Major subdivisions or subheadings of the topic (or important facts that relate to the subject) are connected by lines to the central box and marked '2' (advertisement, prescreening, distribution at study site).
As you go deeper into the subject and uncover another level of information (further subheadings, or individual facts) belonging to the subheadings (level '2'), draw these as lines linked to the subheadings and mark them as level '3'.
Further levels are possible and you can also link different aspects with connecting lines.
The numbers of the levels (1–3 in ➤ Fig. 5.2) are only used to demonstrate the level of headings and are not usually written in a Mind Map.

Free software is available to produce Mind Maps: e.g. FreeMind (freeware) or MindManager (shareware).

5.2 Guidelines for clinical trials

When performing clinical research you have to follow the relevant guidelines. Your institution may have quality assurance guidelines and you may also have to consider Good Clinical Practice.

Good Clinical Practice (GCP) was developed for drug trials and is an international quality standard provided by the International Conference on Harmonization (ICH). The full guideline E6 (R1) is available at www.ich.org or at www.emea.europa.eu. However, as the guideline implies, the principles may also be applied to other clinical investigations (e.g. non pharmaceutical studies) which may have an impact on the safety and well-being of human subjects.

Compliance with these standards provides public assurance that the rights, safety and well-being of trial subjects are protected and that the clinical trial data are credible. The standards are consistent with the principles of the Declaration of Helsinki. The objective of the GCP Guideline is to provide unified standards for the European Union (EU), Japan and the United States to facilitate the mutual acceptance of clinical data by the regulatory authorities in the relevant jurisdictions. The guideline was developed with

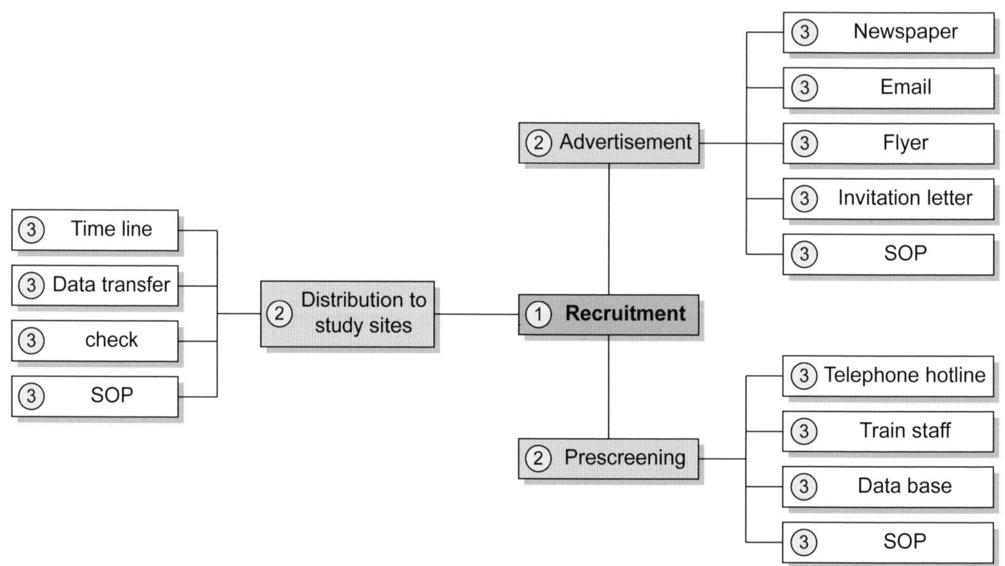

Fig. 5.2 Example of a Mind Map

consideration of the current good clinical practices of the European Union, Japan, and the United States, as well as those of Australia, Canada, the Nordic countries and the World Health Organization (WHO). It must be followed when generating clinical trial data intended to be submitted to regulatory authorities. The principles are displayed in the following box.

Principles of Good Clinical Practice E6 (R1)

- Clinical trials should be conducted in accordance with the ethical principles that have their origin in the Declaration of Helsinki, and that are consistent with GCP and the applicable regulatory requirement(s).
- Before a trial is initiated, foreseeable risks and inconveniences should be weighed against the anticipated benefit for the individual trial subject and society. A trial should be initiated and continued only if the anticipated benefits justify the risks.
- The rights, safety, and well-being of the trial subjects are the most important considerations and should prevail over interests of science and society.
- The available nonclinical and clinical information on an investigational product should be adequate to support the proposed clinical trial.
- Clinical trials should be scientifically sound, and described in a clear, detailed protocol.
- A trial should be conducted in compliance with the protocol that has received prior institutional review board (IRB)/independent ethics committee (IEC) approval/favorable opinion.
- The medical care given to, and medical decisions made on behalf of, subjects should always be the responsibility of a qualified physician or, when appropriate, of a qualified dentist.
- Each individual involved in conducting a trial should be qualified by education, training, and experience to perform his or her respective task(s).
- Freely given informed consent should be obtained from every subject prior to clinical trial participation.
- All clinical trial information should be recorded, handled, and stored in a way that allows its accurate reporting, interpretation and verification.
- The confidentiality of records that can identify subjects should be protected, respecting the privacy and confidentiality rules in accordance with the applicable regulatory requirement(s).
- Investigational products should be manufactured, handled, and stored in accordance with applicable good manufacturing practice (GMP). They should be used in accordance with the approved protocol.
- Systems with procedures that assure the quality of every aspect of the trial should be implemented.

The GCP E6 guideline is divided into the following chapters: investigator (describing qualification and responsibilities), sponsor (describing responsibilities, including financing), clinical trial protocols and protocol amendments, investigators booklet brochure (describing the content), essential documents for the conduct of a trial and the institutional review board/independent ethics committee (describing function, responsibilities and required documents).

5.3 Study management

Commonly more months are spent running a trial than planning it or analyzing its data. Trial management is challenging, especially for beginners, and it is always helpful to work in a team. This chapter will give you an overview of the most important aspects of trial management.

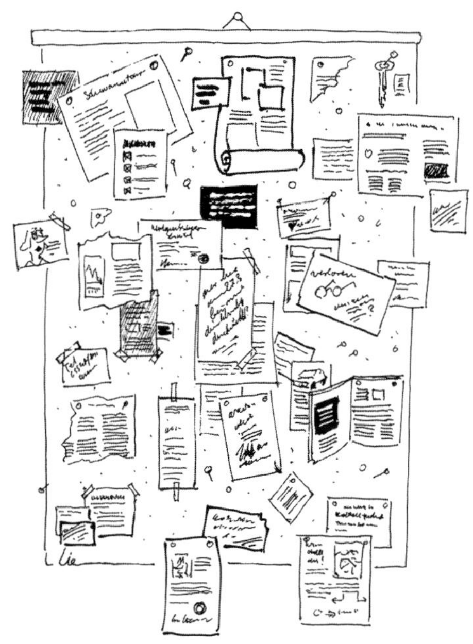

5.3.1 Theoretical background

Timelines and documentation

You have scheduled your study over a certain time period. The schedule should include finances and your personal time involvement. During the planning of a study, parameters that may possibly impact on your time lines are uncertain. It is well known that recruitment often takes longer than planned. Keep this in mind when setting your time lines for the study protocol. However, other aspects cannot be preplanned, for example staff leaving during the study period. You do not need only to plan your time lines you also need to manage them throughout the study with the aim that the study ends as close as possible to the preplanned deadline.

Another important part of study management is the communication within the study team and the documentation of the process and the decisions. For example if you perform a study under particular drug regulations the documentation has to follow the relevant guidelines and will be relatively time consuming. In addition you need to keep in mind that a study is often performed over several years and staff may change. At the end of the study, proper documentation will also be helpful to provide a good overview of what happened during the study and how your results may have been influenced. Other parts of the documentation are required for legal purposes.

!

Standard Operating Procedures

For all procedures within your study you should write **Standard Operating Procedures (SOPs)**. They give written instructions to achieve uniformity of specific processes. They also ensure that trials are conducted and data are generated, documented, and reported in compliance with the study protocol, and the applicable regulatory requirements.
It depends on the type, size and context of your study how detailed these SOPs have to be. What is important is that you have documentation of the responsibilities and processes. A small single center observational study on massage could be done with a few pages of structured notes whereas a drug trial has often more than 100 pages of SOPs in compliance with GCP.

Finances and study team

Support is the basis for any study. You would be hard pressed to do research without a financial budget or the support of staff. When writing your study protocol you included a financial plan. You will now have to check whether it fits the current study situation. The size of your study team depends on the size and the budget of your study. It can range from a single investigator to multiple full time staff. Regardless of the size, all study teams must accomplish similar activities (➤ Table 5.1) and in small studies often one person carries out more than one of these activities.

There are further roles which have to be considered (➤ Table 5.2). GCP demands that in drug trials

Table 5.1 Roles and functions in study teams

Role	Function
Principal investigator (PI)	Main responsible person for the design, conduct, quality and reporting of the study, often an experienced senior researcher
Project coordinator	Day to day management of all study activities
Investigator	A person responsible for the conduct of the clinical trial at a trial site. If a trial is conducted by a team of individuals at a trial site, the investigator is the responsible leader of the team
Research assistant	Carries out study procedures and makes measurements at the study sites; when placed at the study office assists in study management
Data manager	Designs, tests, and implements systems for data entry, -editing and storage, often runs descriptive data analysis
Statistician	Calculates sample size, writes the section on statistical analysis in the study protocol, writes the statistical analysis plan, performs the statistical analysis
Monitor	Person responsible for monitoring the data quality at the study sites
Staff for data entry	Student workers or other staff who enter data

Table 5.2 Further roles and functions

Role	Function
Sponsor	An individual, company, institution, or organization which takes responsibility for the initiation, management, and/or financing of a clinical trial
Sponsor-Investigator	An individual who both initiates and conducts, alone or with others, a clinical trial, and under whose immediate direction the study intervention is administered to a subject. The term only applies to an individual (e.g., it does not include a corporation or an agency). The obligations of a sponsor-investigator include both those of a sponsor and those of an investigator
Steering Committee	The Steering Committee is chaired by an individual who is independent of the investigators who designed and are implementing the trial, in order to provide independent oversight of the study. The Steering Committee will have other independent representation, usually including statistical expertise, and often including lay individuals from either the general public or disease interest groups. Trial investigators may also sit on this committee. The Trial Steering Committee is vested with primary responsibility for the ethical running of the trial
Advisory Board	An advisory board is a body that advises the principal investigator, but does not have authority to make decisions
Independent Data-Monitoring Committee (IDMC) (synonym: Data and Safety Monitoring Board, Monitoring Committee, Data Monitoring Committee)	An independent data-monitoring committee can be established by the sponsor to assess the progress of a clinical trial, the safety data, and the critical efficacy endpoints at suitable intervals, and to make recommendations whether to continue, modify, or stop a trial

the sponsor has to be clearly defined. In investigator initiated trials this role is filled by the principal investigator. In addition to the activities and roles mentioned above external Boards and Committees can be established to strengthen the quality of the results.

Monitoring

Monitoring oversees the progress of a clinical trial, and ensures that it is conducted, recorded, and reported in accordance with the protocol, the SOPs, GCP and the applicable regulatory requirements. Monitoring verifies that the reported trial data are accurate and complete. In multi center trials the monitors are often the main line of communication between the sponsor and the investigator. The monitoring process has to be described in SOPs and after each site visit and other trial-related communication a report which is called monitoring report has to be written by the monitor.

According to the GCP guideline the determination of the extent and nature of monitoring should be based on considerations such as the objective, purpose, design, complexity, blinding, size, and endpoints of the trial. Because many trials are multicenter trials, there usually is a need for on-site monitoring, before, during, and after the trial. This means, for example, that the monitor at the study site compares the data in the CRFs with the source data (e.g. patient clinic record). However, in exceptional circumstances or, for example, in small single center trials central monitoring in conjunction with procedures such as training and meetings of the investigators, and extensive written guidance can assure appropriate conduct of the trial in accordance with GCP without visiting the study sites.

The responsibilities of a monitor are described in detail under point 5.18 on page 26 in the GCP guideline E6 (R1).

5.3.2 Manage your study

You have already managed two phases of your project: the initiation and the planning phase. The next step is to get your study started. Many of these steps such as finances, team building and insuring patients may have already been clarified, however, to be on the safe side, it is better to go through the details again.

The most important steps to manage the execution phase of your study are:

Manage your study	
Step 1	Check your finances
Step 2	Build your team
Step 3	Insure your patients
Step 4	Register your study
Step 5	Arrange day to day study management
Step 6	Organize your material
Step 7	Plan the monitoring
Step 8	Develop a procedure for reporting Adverse Drug Reactions

Step 1: Check your finances

Before you can start your study you have to clarify your finances. Go though each position (see example in the following box) and document the financing of each aspect.

Study staff salaries
- Principal investigator
- Project coordinator
- Research assistant
- Data manager
- Statistician
- Data entry personnel

Study centers (honorary or rent for space)
Intervention (e.g. medication/placebo, pharmacy)
Government and regulatory approval (fees)
Ethical committee approval (fees)
Insurance
Laboratory costs
Printing costs and mailing costs
Travel costs
Monitoring costs
Publication costs

!

You should not start the study if you realize that it does not have enough funding. For example it would be absolutely wrong to reduce the sample size in order to fit the financing since this would be very likely to give you a negative result.

Step 2: Build your team

After you have clarified the finances you should build you team. It makes often sense to start building your team parallel to the financial step, because getting the right staff can be time consuming. However, to implement contracts you usually need the money on the account. The positions of staff within the team including duties and responsibilities should be clarified from the beginning. Before you start your study clarify at the very least who is performing the following activities: principal investigator, project coordinator, research assistant, data manager and statistician. If data entry and monitoring is planned you should also think about these positions. The position of the principal investigator could be an experienced senior researcher. For example this can be the professor where you do your PhD. However, make sure that the principal investigator has the time and energy to be involved in the study since having this position includes huge responsibility for the project. Also keep in mind that depending on your country, principal investigators or investigators at a study site require extra training. This can range between a few hours (e.g. for the investigator at the study site) and 1–2 weeks (e.g. for the principal investigator).

Not everyone has management abilities and although you can get training in management some people are more inclined than others in the application of this skill. If management is not your personal strength, it is highly advisable for the success of your study to draw on another team member (e.g. research assistant) who has this skill and can assist you.

Step 3: Insure your patients

It depends on your study design, your intervention and the context of the study whether and how patients have to be insured. Most IRB/ethics committees require an insurance policy before you get the approval. Better double check before you start your study that you have the appropriate insurance policy and that its content and time lines are up to date.

Step 4: Register your study

You also have to register your study in an open accessible register. The aim behind this is to avoid publication bias. Most journals require registration for publication. You should document the number you receive from the register on your study materials (e.g. study protocol).

Trial registration has to be done after receiving ethical approval and before recruitment.

Different databases are available, such as www.controlled-trials.com/isrctn (costs may apply). A free of charge and frequently used database is www.clinicaltrials.gov.

An additional registration is legally necessary for drug trials. For example in Europe you need to apply for the EudraCT number (eudract.emea.europa.eu/), when you apply for permission from the drug agency. However, you need to keep in mind that this database is not publically accessible and is thus not accepted by journals. This is why you have to additionally register with an open accessible database (➢ Ch. 5.4).

Depending on your country's legal system and the content of your study (drug trial or non-pharmaceutical trial) registration with governmental bodies may also be necessary.

Step 5: Arrange day to day project management

Study management is an accompanying process and you have to formalize at least part of it.

Team meetings

Regular team meetings are the most commonly used instrument and in most studies weekly meetings are held, however, some staff, for example the statistician, may not participate in these frequent meetings. It is important that meetings are structured, and the outcome is documented. This can be done as bullet points or as full text or in a tabular format (➢ Table 5.3).

As you can see not all above described aspects result in an action, some of them are only information points. However they may still be necessary for the management of the study and should thus be documented. It is important that the protocols are stored for easy access by each team member. This may be in an electronic or a paper version.

It makes sense to start each meeting with any open action points from the last meeting before moving to new discussion points. Plan enough time to discuss relevant points, but keep the meetings effective, as their aim is to facilitate the study and not vice versa.

Keeping time lines

Your study has certain time lines fixed in the study protocol. However, often the study starts later than planned; for example, it took longer to get the funding. If this is the case you should define the new time line and also update your study protocol. The main important deadlines are shown in the following list.

- First patient in
- Last patient in
- Last patient out
- Last questionnaire in
- Database closed
- Analysis
- Report
- Publication

One aim of study management is to keep these primary time lines. It is helpful if you also set up secondary time lines. For example, between first pa-

Table 5.3 Example of a structured meeting protocol

Date and time of the meeting: 8.10.2010 14:00–15:00						
Participants: Hilda Scheer, Gerd Doll, Peter Smith, Anne Meyers						
Topic	**Discussion point or information**	**Action**	**Priority**	**Responsible person**	**Deadline**	**Done**
Recruitment	29 patients included	-	-	-	-	-
Recruitment	Too slow	Advertisement in newspaper	high	Peter	15.10.2010	13.10.2010

tient in and last patient in there is often a long time period and you may want to define the date where you would like to have at least 50 % of your patients included. Another example is the publication where you may plan the first draft and the submission date.

Keeping a study record

It is helpful to keep additional non-structured documentation for aspects that can be relevant for data analysis and interpretation of the results. These may be small changes in inclusion or exclusion criteria, for example one inclusion criterion may not have been clearly enough phrased and may have been edited. You can use paper or electronic documentation. You should document all relevant changes and decisions that happen during the study with the date when the changes happen. Decisions are also documented in the meeting protocols, but it would be very time consuming to check all meeting protocols (there can be more than 100) at the end of the study to identify any relevant aspects. Before you start to perform the data analysis you should go through your study records and extract all those aspects which may have an influence.

5

!

Keep also in mind that for relevant changes (e.g. extension of the age group) an amendment of the study protocol is necessary and this will also have to be sent to the IRB/ethics committee.

Writing SOPs

You have to document your processes within the study in a standardized way. This helps to improve the quality of your data. Writing the SOPs for your study is an ongoing process. As soon as a process is defined you should write an SOP for it. It depends on the size of your study (multi-center or single center) and the number of team members how detailed the SOPs have to be.

Keep in mind each study should have at least some SOPs and they should be written as clearly as possible. This means short, well structured and with comprehensible information. Even for a small pilot study you should document at least the responsibilities and the most important processes, e.g. the technique you will use to measure the blood pressure. Some of the information needed for the SOPs may already be in your study protocol.

SOPs may change over time and so different versions may exist. Each SOP should carry a version number, a date and it should be signed by all responsible individuals.

Step 6: Organize your material

You will have recognized by now that planning and conducting a clinical study means developing a large number of documents. These documents need to be organized in a structured and accessible way in which current versions may be easily identified. In addition you have to organize storage of CRFs containing your study data.

!

Also keep in mind that in most countries study documents have to be stored for 10 years after the end of the study.

In larger studies you will have a coordinating trial office and research assistants who will set up your documentation and care for the storage. However in smaller studies you might have to do this yourself. It is helpful to use a obvious system. In the following box you will find some suggestions.

File name with date (e.g. file_year month day)
Footer of each document with file name, version and date
Store older versions in a subfolder and display only the current version in the main folder
Have a clear structure and folder names (see example below)

- STUDY NAME
  - Contracts
  - Study Protocol
  - Investigator booklet/brochure
  - Ethics (correspondence with ethics committee and final vote)
  - Government (correspondence with governmental agencies)
  - Insurance (correspondence with insurance companies)
  - Study registration
  - Investigators (correspondence with study sites)

- Patients (correspondence with patients)
- Patient_CRF
- Physicians_CRF
- Monitoring
- Data management
- Data analysis

Also use a self-explanatory system for the subfolders.

Step 7: Plan the monitoring

You have to decide if you will have monitoring in your study and how much monitoring should be done. This decision depends on the context of the study (e.g. drug trial/non-pharmaceutical trial, single center study/multicenter study) and your budget. Monitoring is resource intensive including human resources and travel expenses. If you don't have your own staff trained in monitoring, the clinical trial center at universities or clinical research organizations (CRO) may provide this service for payment.

If you are in close contact with your study patients, part of the monitoring may be done by a research assistant. For example, if the questionnaires are sent directly by the patient to the coordinating study center the checks for completeness and plausibility of the answers could be done by the personnel of the coordinating study center.

In general monitoring is important to ensure good data quality. Monitoring one hundred percent of the data will be resource intensive, however, so you may instead predetermine the percentage of monitored cases or items. Not all items have the same importance, and you may thus choose to monitor only those which are important for your results (e.g. inclusion and exclusion criteria and main endpoints). If you decide to monitor only a percentage of patients you should choose those patients by a random procedure. If missing items occur – a normal occurrence in clinically based studies – you have to predefine how the monitor or the research assistant in the coordinating study center has to deal with them. One option is to make **queries**. For example, if the birth date of the patient is missing the investigator at the study site will be contacted and asked to provide this information alternatively if the coordinating study center has direct contact with the patient the patient is directly contacted by them.

!

The main aspects of your monitoring should be clarified in your study protocol. In addition the details of the monitoring process have to be clarified in a SOP and after each monitoring a monitoring report has to be written.

Step 8: Develop a procedure how to report adverse reactions

If you run a drug trial you have to report Adverse Drug Reactions that are both serious and unexpected. This reporting hast to be sent to all involved institutions, to the IRB/ethic committees, where required, and to the regulatory authorities. The reports should comply with the applicable regulatory requirements and with the ICH Guideline for Clinical Safety Data Management: Definitions and Standards for Expedited Reporting (www.ich.org).

If you perform a non-pharmaceutical trial it depends on your country's regulations if and where you have to report Adverse Effects.

5.4 Data management

Your study results are based on the data collected during your study. If your data are more complete, reliable and consistent your results will be of higher quality. The data manager should be involved at different stages of the trial: when decisions are made on the format of data collection, during data management and during data analysis. The following chapter will give an overview of the most important aspects of data management during your clinical study.

5.4.1 Theoretical background

GCP defines standards by which trials should be developed, executed, analyzed and reported and the top priority are patients' rights (guideline GCP E6 www.ich.org).

Responsibilities and duties of the data manager:

The data manager is responsible for the design, programming, testing and validating of study databases, the security and integrity of databases, the continuous backup of all databases and the quality control of the data. This also includes generating queries and requesting data from the participating study centers, to organise the data sets and prepare them for analysis.

Data protection

Handling patient data in clinical studies is highly sensitive with regards to data protection. Considering patient confidentiality there are different types of data, personalized data, anonymous data and pseudonymous data. **Anonymous data** means that there is no way to connect the data with a person. In most clinical studies you have **personalized data** which may be name, address and telephone number of patient. Often these data are stored only at the study site where the physician has direct contact with the patient. There may be exceptions where the data are additionally stored in the coordinating study center, such as if direct contact between the research assistant and the patient is required, for example, to assess the outcome by telephone interviews. If you store personalized data, e.g. in a **study management database,** you have to take the data protection requirements into account. Besides the personalized data you will have **pseudonymous data**. For each patient an identifier (ID) is created and this is used instead of the name. The code list connecting the name with the ID has to be stored in a safe place with restricted and monitored access. This may be a paper or an electronic database (e.g. the study management database) on a secure server. As long as the code list is secure the **CRF databases** which include the study results and use only the ID can be handled without data protection problems.

!

Your trial has to follow the local and regional laws for data protection in your country. To protect patient's confidentiality, databases that contain personalized data must be stored on secure servers, with restricted and (password) secured access.

Databases

Databases for clinical studies fulfil different objections. They are helpful for managing your trial data which includes registration, randomization and follow-up management of the study participants. In addition they are used to enter the values obtained during the study. It depends on your study and the context how many databases you will develop, but it is useful to create different databases: **study management data bases** and **CRF databases.** For CRF databases it is helpful to develop different databases, for example, for patient and practitioner CRF. Data from the same source, but from different evaluation time points should be stored in different tables because this makes the work of your data manager more efficient. For example data from an earlier follow up time point will be available earlier which means that the file of this table can be cleaned and finalized before the files of the later time points are cleaned. At the end of a trial the schedule is always tight and everything which can be finalized before final deadlines will help to keep your time line.

It is a matter of security and data quality that the person who is working with databases has proper knowledge of the used software. If this is not the case you may create invalid data or even lose it. There is a range of software for data management available, e.g. Microsoft Access, Microsoft Excel, Oracle, SQL Server, SPSS and Stata.

All computer databases consist of one or more tables in which the rows correspond to records and the columns to items. For example in a very simple study on hypertension you will only have one CRF database with one row for each patient, identified with the ID, and a column for each item, e.g. age, sex, years at school, duration of disease, systolic blood pressure at baseline, diastolic blood pressure at baseline, systolic blood pressure at 3 months, diastolic blood pressure at 3 months (➢ Table 5.4).

If the data are limited to a single table, this data can be easily entered into a spreadsheet (e.g. Excel or SPSS). However if you have several treatments and want to document the information from the treatments continuously (date, duration, number of needles, side effects) a **relational database** is

Table 5.4 Simplified data for a pilot study on acupuncture for hypertension with 10 subjects and a pre-post comparison

ID	age_y	sex	school_y	disease_y	systol_t0	diastol_t0	systol_t1	diastol_t1
101	54	F	10	7	157	103	145	96
102	47	M	12	12	160	100	150	100
103	43	M	10	3	149	90	145	90
104	37	F	12	4	165	110	140	80
105	65	M	10	12	162	95	142	90
106	44	F	10	5	157	92	158	100
107	31	F	10	2	163	92	150	90
108	37	F	12	3	154	80	130	80
109	34	M	12	2	166	97	140	79
110	45	F	12	8	155	100	160	90

Table 5.5 Relational database with two tables. In the table 'patients' each row corresponds to one patient. In table 'treatments' each row corresponds to one treatment. Treatments from different patients' are documented continuously. Since a patient can have more than one treatment the relation between the table 'patients' and the table 'treatments' is one-to-many

Table_patients

ID	age_y	sex	school_y	disease_y	systol_t0	diastol_t0	systol_t1	diastol_t1
101	54	f	10	7	157	103	145	96
102	47	m	12	12	160	100	150	100
103	43	m	10	3	149	90	145	90
104	37	f	12	4	165	110	140	80
105	65	m	10	12	162	95	142	90
106	44	f	10					
107	31	f	10					
108	37	f	12					
109	34	m	12					
110	45	f	12					

Table_treatments

n_treat	*ID*	*dur_min*	*n_needles*	*safety*
1	**101**	30	10	1
2	102	32	15	1
3	**101**	28	10	1
4	107	30	14	1
5	103	29	15	1
6	106	31	13	2
7	**101**	32	12	1
8	105	30	16	1

useful. In this kind of database the relation between the patient and the table of treatments is one-to-many (➤ Table 5.5). Relational databases can be helpful for the study management database.

!

For CRF databases relational databases have the advantage that the information is comprehensive, but redundant storage is eliminated. However, their limitation is that the data must be reorganized, because for the statistical software you need the data for each patient in one row. If you are not an experienced data manager a simplified database can be more suitable.

Data dictionary, variable name and value labels

In a data table each column has a name, a data type and a definition. In the table 'patients' the column 'age_y' stands for the variable 'age' it is a 'numeric' field and is defined as 'age of the patient measured in years'.

The **data dictionary** is part of your software and makes the column definitions explicit. The data dictionary can be a table with rows representing the variables (fields) and columns for the field name, field type and field description and a set of allowed values.

The **variable (or field) name** should give a short but clear identification. You can use the full word for short names (e.g. age) and common abbreviations for longer words (e.g. Pat_ID for patient identification).

The **value labels** are descriptions on the different possible responses that you type into the database. For example you may have decided to use the value label 1 for 'yes'. It is very important to remember your coding for the various answers. For example if you want to calculate something from a 5 year old file and you have no value labels for 1 and 2 which are in the column sex, you would be in trouble. Also for more obvious values such as pain on the VAS it can be helpful to put additional information for the value label for example the scale of measurement (cm or mm).

Setting allowed values is helpful to reduce typing errors during data entry, e.g. for the variable 'sex' only '1' and '2' should be allowed. Typing in a '3' would then be rejected by the software (➤ Table 5.6).

The questionnaire on page 117 will use the examples from the chapter 'outcomes' and show how the responses for these questions will be transferred into a database.

Table 5.6 Commonly used field types

Field type	Explanation
ID	Most data entry programs will automatically assign consecutive numbers, so if you have your own patient IDs you should create a further variable, e.g. add the patient name with the pat_code
Numeric	Numeric variables can be whole numbers or decimals, (you can specify how many digits you will accept after the comma), and should be used for all continuous variables e.g. systolic blood pressure or pain on the VAS and all categorical variables e.g. gender (1 = male, 2 = female) or pain ratings (1 = no pain, 2 = light pain, 3 = moderate pain, 4 = strong pain)
Logical (yes/no)	Logical variables are entered as 'yes' or 'no'. For statistical analysis it will be necessary to recode the variable to a numeric value. However they can be more convenient for data management than a numeric field
Date	Date variables are only used for specific dates (e.g. birth date, enrolment date). You can use them to calculate intervals between the dates
Text	Text variables allow you to enter open ended comments made by the patient or practitioner. The text responses cannot be analyzed statistically unless you categorize them into responses with certain numbers. However, it is better to enter the free text data together with the numeric data instead of going back into the questionnaires, if the data are needed later

5.4.2 Manage your data

Being a good data manager or having a good data manager in your team is fundamental for a clinical trial. The practical steps explained here mainly focus on paper and pencil documentation, where you have to develop databases and enter the data manually from the CRFs.

The most important steps for successful data management are:

Manage your data	
Step 1	Creating variable names and value labels
Step 2	Developing your databases
Step 3	Collecting your data
Step 4	Entering your data
Step 5	Looking after your data
Step 6	Cleaning the data file
Step 7	Preparing your data for analysis

1. How old are you?

Please fill in your age in years:
Database: field name 'age', numeric variable, no digits after comma, allowed values 18–65, definition: age of the patient

2. How severe was your average pain in the last 7 days?

Please mark your average pain intensity on the line
No pain I--I maximum conceivable pain
Database: field name 'VAS_t0', numeric variable, no digits behind comma, allowed values 0–100, definition: pain at baseline measured on the VAS

3. Have you ever had an operation on your spine?

1) Yes □
2) No □
Database: field name 'OP_t0', numeric variable, no digits after comma, allowed values 1 and 2 (1 = yes, 2 = no), definition: previous spine operation

4. Which of the following symptoms are you currently experiencing?

a) Headache yes □ no □
Database: field name 'head_t0', numeric variable, no digits after comma, allowed values 1 and 2 (1 = yes, 2 = no), definition: current symptom headache
b) Dizziness yes □ no □
Database: field name 'dizzi_t=', numeric variable, no digits after comma, allowed values 1 and 2 (1 = yes, 2 = no), definition: current symptom dizziness
c) Cough yes □ no □
Database: field name 'cough_t0', numeric variable, no digits after comma, allowed values 1 and 2 (1 = yes, 2 = no), definition: current symptom cough
d) Sore throat yes □ no □
Database: field name 'throat_t0', numeric variable, no digits after comma, allowed values 1 and 2 (1 = yes, 2 = no), definition: current symptom sore throat
e) Back pain yes □ no □
Database: field name 'back_t0 numeric variable, no digits after comma, allowed values 1 and 2 (1 = yes, 2 = no), definition: current symptom back pain
f) Other: ____________________________________
Database: field name 'othersym_t0, text variable, definition: further symptoms

5. Osteopathy is effective for pain treatment

1) Strongly agree □
2) Agree □
3) Mildly agree □
4) Disagree □
5) Strongly disagree □
Database: field name 'believe_t0', numeric variable, no digits after comma, allowed values 1–5 (1 = strongly agree, 2 = agree, 3 = mildly agree, 4 = disagree, 5 = strongly disagree), definition: believe whether osteopathy is effective for pain treatment

Step 1: Creating variable names and value labels

As a first step you should get an overview of the variables which you evaluate during your study.

! You should create a field name for each variable, a field type, value labels, write the field description and define the allowed values. If you have variables which are evaluated at different time points, for example pain measured on the VAS at baseline und after 3 months, the variable names have to be different for each time point (e.g. (VAS_0 and VAS_3 or VAS_t0 and VAS_t1)

5

It is very helpful to take an empty questionnaire and to write the field name, value labels and allowed values beside the questions, before you transfer this information into the data dictionary of your software. You may keep this questionnaire as **'annotated CRF'**. This will be useful for the interpretation of your data analysis output.

Step 2: Developing the study databases

The development of the study databases takes some time and should be started as soon as the details are determined. You have to choose the software and if you work with an established research group it is better to use whatever database program the others in your group are using which will help you if you run into problems.

Study management database

Before you start to include patients in your study you should establish your study management database. For example you can use this for the registration of your patients, the communication with the study centers and with patients (if needed), the management of the follow up and the query process. You can include a randomization tool if needed, but you will need to ensure that the person who allocates the patients to the groups has no access to the randomization sequence and no influence on the result of the randomization. If you have to send materials to the study centers you can use this database to monitor the process. It is also a useful instrument to provide regular standard reports, for example, on aspects like number of recruited patients per center, number of patients recruited in week 10, number of drop outs, etc.

!

If the study management database contains personal data of patients (e.g. name, address) it has to be stored on a secure server with restricted access (e.g. password protection and monitored access to password and database). This database must be totally unconnected with the CRF databases, which contain the data from the study evaluation.

The following box provides examples of information which can be documented in the study management database.

- If needed, patients' personalized data: name, address, telephone number, email, ID, treatment group
- Contact data of study centers: practitioners, address, telephone number, email, ID
- Communication with patients: date, topic, decision
- Communication with study centers: data, topic decision
- Materials: dates when sent out
- Follow-up questionnaires: dates when sent out, dates for incoming questionnaires, dates for reminders
- Queries: dates when sent out, dates when solved
- Drop outs with reason
- Notes

CRF databases

The CRF databases contain your research data (as documented by patients and/or practitioners). The design and number of databases and tables depend on the complexity of the collected data. If your study has only a small number of patients, (e.g. up to 100), two measurement time points and a limited number of variables (e.g. up to 30), you can enter your data directly into the spreadsheet of a statistics software (e.g. SPSS).

If you have a larger trial, more variables and more measurement time points orientation in a spreadsheet would be difficult and data entry errors are more likely to occur. In this case you need more complex databases (different tables and perhaps a relational database). Plan the structure of your database before you start entering data into it.

The data entry will be more convenient if you create forms which look similar to the questionnaire.

!

Keep in mind that in all tables the data of each patient has the unique patient ID and be careful that you don't mix this up with the automatically generated ID in the software.

Validity of databases

Once you have finalized the design of your databases it is helpful to test them. This is done by data entry and running the main query procedures. Regular backups of your data are required and you have to develop a backup procedure. This procedure has to be described in a SOP.

If you run a drug trial and follow GCP you must validate your data base. Document how and with which results you have tested the validity of your databases. The program should run under usual circumstances as well as under difficult circumstances. You will need an **audit trail**. This is an automated process which provides a means for tracing items of data for each processing step. It monitors and documents changes. The following information has to be recorded: date of change, identity of person who made the change, old value, new value and name of the variable. However, for this you really need a professional data manager.

Step 3: Collecting your data

Paper and pencil data collection

In most studies data collection is spread over a long period of time, often years, mainly using paper and pencil for documentation. For the quality of the data it is important that the data are collected at predefined time points and that the person who is responsible for the completeness, consistency and reliability of the data (monitor or research assistant) checks the data as promptly as possible. This can be at the study site (e.g. in a practitioner practice) or centrally in the study organization center if the patients send their questionnaires directly to the coordinating study center.

!

For inconsistent data or missing data you should develop clear SOPs where you define for each variable the action necessary.

For example if the age is missing or the VAS for pain was not marked, the practitioner has to be contacted and asked to contact the patient. If you have direct patient contact you may contact the patient yourself. For another, less important variable (e.g. therapies the patient is interested in) you may accept the missing data without further action. The SOP can be in the format of a table (➤ Table 5.7).

Electronic data capture

If you collect your data using electronic CRFs you can do this offline through on-screen forms or online through web pages. This eliminates the data entry, but needs sophisticated data entry forms which already include direct checks for completeness, plausibility and consistency of the data entered. In addition, a source document should be printed directly. This can be used for monitoring.

5

Step 4: Entering your data

After your CRFs have been checked for completeness and plausibility and all queries are clarified, the data can be entered into the database. This is an important step, which needs standardization to ensure correct data entry. This means that anyone who enters the data (e.g. research assistant or student workers) must be trained and the data entry follows the SOPs. Here again for each variable clear actions have to be predefined. For example for many validated questionnaires (e.g. SF-36) you will find clear advice

Table 5.7 SOP for the patients' baseline questionnaire

SOP for the patients' baseline questionnaire Version 1.0_10.9.2010			
Question number	Variable	Options	Action
1	Age	Missing	Check patient record or contact practitioner/patient
2	Gender	Missing	Check patient record or contact practitioner/patient
3	School education	Missing	Contact practitioner/patient
		two responses marked	Take the higher education
4	Pain VAS	Missing	Send copy of questionnaire to patient/practitioner and ask for completion
		Two marks	Send copy of questionnaire to patient/practitioner and ask for clarification
5	Belief in acupuncture	Missing	No action (leave as missing)

in the hand book or publication how to deal with missing data or double responses.

You have to ensure the quality of your data entry procedure. One standard method to control the data quality is a **double data entry**. This is needed for drug trials which follow the GCP guidelines. A cheaper option is **a visual check of a random sample** where the entered data is compared with the data in the questionnaire (e.g. 10 %, 30 % or 50 % of the data entered by each person). Both the second data entry as well as the visual check should be done by a different person from the one who entered the data the first time. Also **programmed data checks** on plausibility can be used to get a feeling for the quality of the data entry.

Double data entry is still the best way to get accurate data. Two methods could be used. The first uses two independent files for both data entries and compares them. The data where you find differences will be listed and you have to check the paper CRF for the correct version and edit the main file. Another option is that both files are connected, and when the second person enters the data it checks directly whether the entered value differs from the previously entered value (key-to-key verification). In case of differences the correct value will be determined from the paper CRF.

5

!

Data entry is time consuming, has to be standardized and the quality has to be controlled.

Step 5: Looking after your data

Data management is a process that is linked to data entry and continues throughout the whole study. You will report on study progress (e.g. recruitment of patients) from the study management data base and also on the data entry progress from the CRF data base. You have to do database **queries** to sort and filter the data and to produce reports. A query can join data from two or more tables, display only selected fields and filter for data that meet certain criteria. Queries can also calculate values based on raw data fields from the tables, for example the time period between recruitment and end of treatment from the dates of both time points.

You may also import data from other sources, e.g. hospital databases into your database. However this should only be only done if you have figured out how to do it in a valid way.

!

Keep in mind that you have to define the data management processes in SOPs and you have to keep a proper documentation of the structure of tables, queries and forms (program code).

Step 6: Cleaning your files

Cleaning your files means that you identify and correct errors in the data which have been entered into the databases.

!

Before you start cleaning your data you should save your raw data and store it clearly labelled (e.g. table_patients_raw_final_101122). You can then take a copy of the file and start your plausibility checks.

The data base should be queried for missing values and outliers (values that lie within the range of allowed values but at the outer range).

For example if a 10 year old has a weight entry of 60 kg it should be queried. You also have to decide how missing data should be coded (e.g. –1 or 999). Missing values, outliers, inconsistencies, and other data problems are clarified using queries. They are communicated to the study staff, who can respond to them by checking original source documents, interviewing the patient, or repeating the measurement if possible.

!

If the study relies on paper sources, any changes in the questionnaires should be highlighted, dated and signed. Electronic databases should maintain an audit trail.

If data are collected by different investigators from different sites the values for the mean and median should be compared across investigators and sites. Substantial differences can indicate a systematic difference in measurement and data collection and should be further investigated.

You should give higher priority to more important variables. For example, in a randomized back pain trial the most important variables are the outcome measures and no errors should be tolerated. In contrast errors in other variables, such as consultations dates, may not substantially affect the results of your study.

!

After errors are identified and corrected, the query procedure should be repeated until very few important errors are identified. At that point the database should be closed and labelled accordingly. After closure no further changes should be permitted even if further errors are identified.

Step 7: Preparing your data for analysis

The clean file has to be converted into a format which can be used in statistics software (e.g. SPSS, SAS). This includes labelling of variables and response values.

Analyzing data often requires creating new, derived variables based on the raw field values. For example for most validated questionnaires you have to calculate values for subscales. You can find information on how to do this in the handbook or publications of the various questionnaires.

5.5 Case studies

In this chapter we will not show each step for the three case studies, but instead we will provide you with a summary comment on each study. This will provide information on how much study and data management will be necessary for each study type.

Case study 1: Uncontrolled observational study (pilot study)

Case study 1 is a descriptive, observational study without control group evaluating one treatment with special acupuncture needles that are left in situ for 7 days, an uncommon procedure but one frequently used by one particular acupuncturist.

This is a small and descriptive single center observational study on a non pharmaceutical intervention. The investigator has limited human resources and no external funding to run the study. In view of the type of intervention and the study setting, study management and data management can be reduced to a minimal standard focussing on receiving complete and valid data. SOP could be reduced to core standards such as responsibilities and the most important study processes and a simple data base (e.g. SPSS spreadsheet) could be used to enter the study data. Nevertheless, it is important to adhere to data protection laws. Although in most countries this counts as an observational study, ethical approval is needed and clarification is needed whether patients have to be insured for the study.

Case study 2: Randomized double-blind placebo-controlled study

Case study 2 is an efficacy study. The objective of this randomized controlled trial is to evaluate whether an herbal medicine product containing an extract of Harpagophytum procumbens (Devil's claw) and given for two months is more effective than placebo in patients with chronic low back pain.

This is a multi-center drug trial and study and data management have to reflect a high standard. This trial needs reasonable funding to provide for adequate human resources, to follow the ICH-GCP guidelines and to take all regulatory aspects into account.

Case study 3: Pragmatic randomized study comparing three groups

Case study 3 is a comparative effectiveness study in a usual care setting. The objective of this pragmatic randomized three-armed trial is to evaluate whether acupuncture treatment or yoga in addition to usual care is more effective in the treatment of patients with chronic low back pain than usual care alone and whether acupuncture is more effective than Yoga in this context.

This is a large multi-center pragmatic study and to produce valid results the study and the data management should be of high quality. The paragraphs of ICH-GCP which can be transferred to non-pharmaceutical trials should be fulfilled.

CHAPTER

6 Data analysis

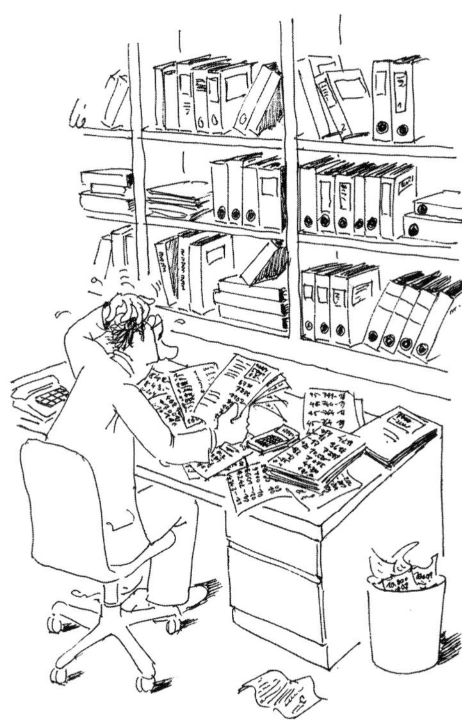

6.1 Analysing your own data step by step

After you have collected your data and cleaned your file it can be analyzed. ➢ Chapter 3 of this book gave an introduction into basics statistics. Here we want to guide you step by step through your statistical analysis. You will have defined the main aspects of your statistical analysis already in the study protocol (➢ Ch. 4.2). Before analyzing your data, you should write a '**statistical analysis plan (SAP)**' which contains more details about the analysis than the study protocol does. The SAP defines the populations to be analysed, and the primary and all secondary endpoints and describes all planned statistical analyses that will be used for each of the endpoints (including sensitivity analyses and the procedures for dealing with missing values). A short example for a statistical analysis plan is given in Case Study Two. If you define your analysis before performing it, you can call this a '**predefined statistical analysis**'. All further analyses which were not predefined are so called '**post hoc analyses**'.

There are seven main steps for data analysis. We will run through them step by step and use the case studies as examples. Step 1–4 help to prepare your statistical analysis and the decisions should be documented in the SAP. Step 5 shows the actual analysis and Steps 6 and 7 the reporting of the data.

Statistical analysis	
Step 1	Define the analysis populations and the handling of missing values
Step 2	Identify the different types of variable
Step 3	Clarify what you can calculate from your data
Step 4	Choose suitable statistical methods
Step 5	Perform the statistical analysis
Step 6	Decide how you will present your results
Step 7	Interpret your results and conclude

6.1.1 Step 1: Define the analysis populations and the handling of missing values

Remember there are different kinds of analysis populations such as ITT and PP (➢ Ch. 3.7). If this is a study evaluating the superiority of one intervention compared to another, you have to use an intention-to-treat-analysis. This should already be clarified in the study protocol. In the **intention-to-treat-analysis** you include all patients that were randomized. You might decide in advance that you include only those patients that received at least one treatment, but you will have to make this transparent. In addition to the ITT analysis you could conduct a per-protocol-analysis (this would be called **secondary analysis**). For the per-protocol-analysis (PP) you have to predefine the relevant aspects of the protocol, such as a minimum number of treatment sessions attended or absence of prohibited co-interventions. These per- protocol criteria should define a population of patients who had an optimal treatment according to your treatment protocol. Be careful that your criteria are not too narrow, to ensure that you will have enough patients left in this population. The criteria for the PP population have to be documented in the statistical analysis plan before you start the analysis.

You also have to define how you would like to deal with the **missing values** in your data set. Missing values means that no data are present for the variable in the current time point. This is a common occurrence, because not all patients complete their questionnaires or show up for all appointments. Methods such as last value carried forward are easy to use whereas other methods (e.g. multiple imputations) use statistical procedures and should be done by a statistician. You can decide to do the primary analysis already with imputed data for missing values or you perform first the primary analysis including only the available data and afterwards you perform a sensitivity analysis where the missing data will be imputed.

6.1.2 Step 2: Identify the different types of variable

In our case studies we use different variables, including the average pain in the last 7 days measured on a Visual Analogue Scale (VAS), back function, quality of life (SF-36), expectations of the patient and blinding during the study. Remember that we have different types of variable and that the way we analyze and display them differs for the different types (➤ Ch. 3.2 and ➤ Table 6.1). Identify this for each of your variables.

Table 6.1 Examples for variables

Variable	Category	Subcategory	Comment
Age (in years)	continuous		
Age groups (< 40, 40–60, > 60)	categorical	ordinal	
Gender	categorical	nominal, dichotomous	
VAS (Visual Analogue Scale 0–100)	continuous		
SF-36 (quality of life)	categorical	ordinal	summary score analyzed as continuous
Back function	categorical	ordinal	summary score analyzed as continuous
Satisfaction with treatment (very high, high, moderate, low, very low)	categorical	ordinal	
Expectation (either: very high, high, moderate, low, very low or: high/low)	categorical	ordinal, dichotomous	

6.1.3 Step 3: Clarify what you can calculate from your data

After each variable is identified you need to clarify how you analyze and display it. This depends not only on the type of variable (continuous or categorical), but also on the distribution (normal or non-normal) (➤ Ch. 3.2). Tests to check for normally distributed data exist, but they are usually quite conservative and often of limited use. Thus, it is often better to graphically display your continuous data in a histogram to get an impression whether the distribution looks approximately normal. ➤ Table 6.2 gives an overview of the various options for displaying data.

Table 6.2 Possible results and options for displaying the variables of case study 1

Variable	Possible results	Display options
Continuous		
VAS, back function, quality of life	Describe the average and the spread Check if normally distributed*: For normal distribution → mean and standard deviation or standard error and/or CI For non-normal distribution → median and interquartile range (25 % and 75 %) For cost data → mean and standard deviation	Text, table or figure (for median and interquartile range use box plots)
Categorical		
Ordinal (blinding, treatment success)	Calculate the frequency of the response for each category in numbers and percentages	Text, a frequency table or a bar graph
Dichotomous (expectation)	Calculate frequencies and proportions	Text or table

* Normally distributed variable → the histogram is bell shaped, non-normally distributed variable → the histogram is skewed, in this case the mean and the median are substantially different from each other and the standard deviation is as big as or bigger than the mean

6.1.4 Step 4: Choose suitable statistical methods

Before starting your statistical analysis you have to choose suitable methods. The appropriate statistical procedure depends on the following questions:

- the type of variable
- whether you are comparing means or proportions
- the number of observations (e.g. measurement time points, or groups) you want to compare

Tables will give some guidance for choosing the appropriate statistical tests or statistical models.

Statistical analysis plan (SAP)

The SAP is a document which extends your study protocol and has to be finalized before analyzing the data. It is based on the study protocol, but provides more detail on the statistical analysis and includes information on:

- Hypotheses
- Analysis population
- Handling of missing data
- Primary and all secondary outcome measures including measurement time points
- Statistical methods for descriptive analyses
- Statistical methods for primary confirmatory analysis
- Statistical analysis for secondary outcome measures and analyses
- Responsibilities
- The final SAP has a date, a version number and is signed by the statistician and the principle investigator

Descriptive analysis

The descriptive analysis summarizes your data. Results will be summarized as mean values, standard deviations, and 95 %-confidence intervals; medians, quartiles, value ranges for continuous data, and frequencies and percentages for categorical data.

Confirmatory analysis (testing the hypothesis)

The confirmatory analysis is the analysis for your primary endpoint and tests your study hypothesis. In your statistical analysis plan you can predefine most tests, however, you do not know in advance whether your data are normally distributed or skewed. For example, in the statistical analysis plan you could write, 'if the data for low back pain intensity are normally distributed we will use an unpaired t-test, if it is not normally distributed we will use Wilcoxon rank sum test'.

The ➢ tables 6.3 and 6.4 can help orientate you when choosing the appropriate statistical test.

In making the final decision you need to know the distribution of your data. However, you only see this during the analysis stage using graphical techniques such as a histogram (➢ Fig. 6.1) or specific statistical tests.

6

Table 6.3 Statistical tests for comparing two observations (two group or two measurement time points)

Variable	Independent observations of different patients	Dependent (repeated) observations of the same patients
Comparing means		
Continuous variables (e.g. blood pressure in mmHg)		
Normally distributed	Unpaired t-test	Paired t-test
Not normally distributed	Wilcoxon rank-sum test	Wilcoxon signed rank test
Comparing proportions or other categories (categorical variables)		
Dichotomous variables (e.g. gender)	Chi-squared test	McNemar's test
Dichotomous variables if small sample size (i.e. expected frequency of any cell < 5)	Fisher's exact test	(exact) McNemar's test
Nominal with more than 2 values (e.g. ethnicity)	Chi-square test	Bowker's test of symmetry
Ordinal variables (e.g. age groups)	Mann-Whitney test (= Wilcoxon rank-sum test)	Wilcoxon signed rank test

Table 6.4 Statistical test for multiple observations (more than 2 groups or more than two measurement time points)

Variable	Independent observations of different patients	Dependent (repeated) observations of the same patients
Categorical variables		
Dichotomous variable	Chi-squared test	Cochrans' Q
Ordinal variable	Kruskal-Wallis test	Friedman test
Continuous variables		
Normally distributed	ANOVA	Repeated measures ANOVA
Not normally distributed	Kruskal-Wallis test	Friedman test

6

➢ Figure 6.1 shows that in this example the pain data (measured on the VAS) are perfectly normally distributed (i.e. bell shaped). In reality the distribution is often a little skewed, but you are still on the safe side if you calculate the mean and standard deviation and you can use the unpaired t-test to compare two groups. But keep in mind that this could be different for other variables.

Multiple testing

If you define more than one primary endpoint in your study protocol you should clarify how you will adjust your analysis accordingly in your SAP (➢ Ch. 3)

You will usually perform many statistical tests for the baseline characteristics of your groups and for your secondary endpoints after treatment. It is very important to distinguish between your primary and secondary endpoints and to describe all comparisons for the secondary endpoints as exploratory. It is also of note that some statisticians argue that testing for baseline differences in randomized trials makes no sense, because, as a result of the process of randomization, baseline differences can only occur by chance.

6.1.5 Step 5: Perform the statistical analysis

If you intend to do the analysis by yourself, it is important that you plan enough time for this and that you familiarize yourself with the software that you will be using. Here are some suggestions for your analysis:

Use standard software for statistical analysis and become fully conversant with this software.

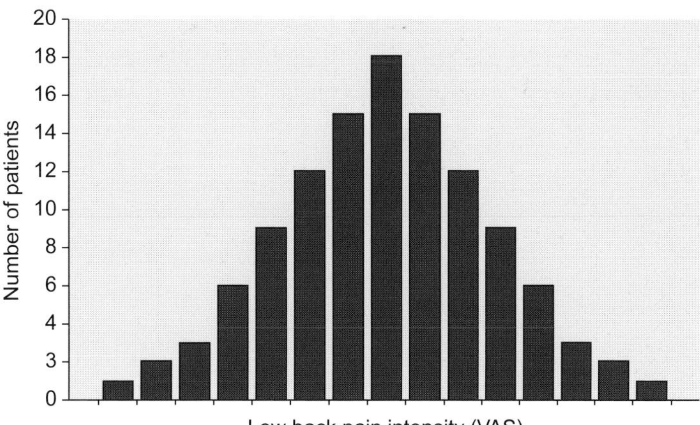

Fig. 6.1 Histogram showing an ideal distribution of the VAS values for pain intensity after 8 weeks

Check the data and the results for plausibility (Is this what you expected? Does it fit with the context of the available scientific information? For example, if you have diastolic blood pressure values of 20 mm Hg, this is implausible and you will need to find the error in your analysis or data).

Recalculate the important results once or twice (e.g. the primary outcome and the main secondary outcomes).

Document your statistical analysis by making notes and saving your files clearly labeled and well sorted. If, later on, you write a report or a publication, it should be clear which analysis file was used for each of the various results.

6.1.6 Step 6: Decide how you will present your results

The presentation of your study results should be clear and comprehensive. This means that the reader should get all the information necessary for interpreting the study results. There are two main presentation types: journal publication ('paper') and report. Journal publications are quite short, whereas reports provide comprehensive information about your study. It could be very helpful to read some papers or reports of authors who have done similar studies. To display your data you can choose between text, figures and tables. Make sure that you don't present the same result in two ways (e.g. in a table and a figure). Tables are usually the most comprehensive way to display lots of data in a small space, whereas figures can be helpful to highlight important results. You can use examples from other publications or reports to plan how you present your data.

6.1.7 Step 7: Interpret your results and draw your conclusions

After you have performed the analysis and displayed your results, you have to interpret them and come to one or more conclusions. Be careful that your conclusions are clearly based on your study question, the statistical methods and the results and that they take any potential flaws or limitations of your study into account.

6.2 Case studies

The three case studies will be used to provide examples for the different steps of the data analysis process. The data analysis of a study depends on many parameters and could vary according to these parameters. Please take into account that for the case studies given here the analysis presented is one option and other options may also be suitable. Because of this it is important that you predefine your analysis before you conduct it, to prevent 'playing around' with your data to produce favorable results.

Case study 1: Uncontrolled observational study (pilot study)

Case study 1 is a descriptive, observational study without control group evaluating a treatment with special acupuncture needles left in situ for 7 days, an uncommon procedure but one frequently used by one particular acupuncturist.

Step 1: Define the analysis population

For the primary analysis, an intention to treat analysis is chosen including all patients who were included into the study and who provided at least baseline data.

Steps 2 and 3: Identify the different types of variable and clarify what you can calculate from your data

In this study you have continuous and categorical variables. The VAS, for example, is a continuous variable and you can display means or mean changes (e.g. between baseline and two months) with SD or 95 % CI. Gender will be analyzed as a categorical variable resulting in numbers and percentages for each category. Although the back function questionnaire (HFAQ) and the quality of life questionnaire (SF-36) are categorical variables the summary scores are usually analyzed using statistics for continuous data and presenting means or mean changes.

Steps 4 and 5: Choose suitable statistical procedures and perform the statistical analysis

This is an exploratory study and you can use simple statistics (e.g. two-sided paired t-test for continuous variables or McNemar's test for categorical variables) or you can ask a statistician to perform a more complex analysis such as multiple measurements ANOVA which is appropriate for more than one follow up time point. In addition you can compare the results of the different outcomes to discuss and identify suitable outcomes for a future larger study. An example of a short description of your statistical analysis could be: 'The statistical analysis is primarily descriptive, and the statistical significance of changes between baseline and follow up is determined on an exploratorybasis (repeated measures ANOVA). The primary analysis will include all available data and in a further sensitivity analysis missing data will be replaced by the last value carried forward method.'

Step 6: Decide how to present your results

Results can be displayed in text, tables or figures. For example: A total of 40 patients (mean age 57.2 ± 7.8 years) were included in our study. Two thirds (67 %) were female and the average disease duration was 12.5 ± 10.7 years. Approximately one third (36 %) had acupuncture treatment before and 77 % had used analgesics in the past six months. The average pain intensity on the 100 mm VAS in the last seven days decreased from 61.1 ± 12.1 to 36.5 ± 27.4 mm after two months, see figure 1, $p < 0.001$) and this effect was nearly maintained for 12 months (➤ Fig. 6.2). Similar improvement was found for other parameters such as back function and quality of life (➤ Table 6.5).

Step 7: Interpret your results and conclude

Patients suffering from chronic low back pain who received a single acupuncture treatment with needles retained for seven days had less back pain, better back function and a higher quality of life after two, six and 12 months compared to baseline. To evaluate whether this effect is caused by the acupuncture technique investigated, a randomized controlled study would be necessary.

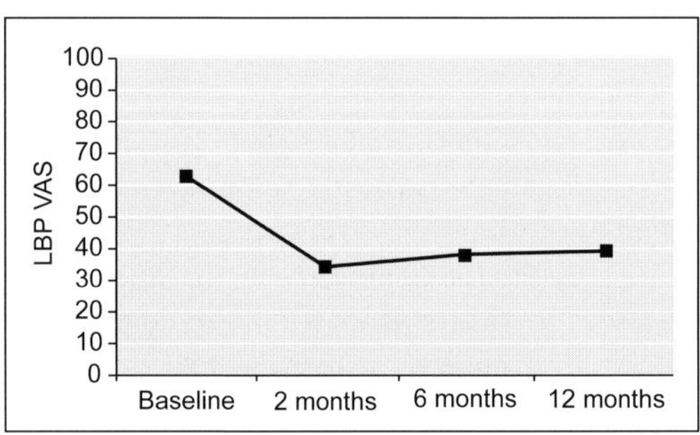

Fig. 6.2 The course of low back pain intensity over 12 months. Mean values and standard deviations (LBP = Low Back Pain, VAS = Visual Analogue Scale)

Table 6.5 Outcome after 2, 6 and 12 months

	Baseline mean ± SD	2 months mean ± SD	6 months mean ± SD	12 months mean ± SD
Back function (HFAQ)	56.1 ± 17.4	66.3 ± 18.8	66.1 ± 20.0	59.9 ± 20.1
SF-36 Physical health	32.5 ± 7.9	41.0 ± 9.9	38.9 ± 9.2	38.9 ± 10.0
SF-36 Mental Health	48.2 ± 10.3	49.9 ± 9.8	49.2 ± 10.4	49.9 ± 10.7

LBP = Low Back Pain, VAS = Visual Analogue Scale

Case study 2: Randomized double-blind placebo-controlled study

Case study 2 is an efficacy study. The objective of this randomized controlled trial is to evaluate whether an herbal medicine product containing an extract of Harpagophytum procumbens (Devil's claw) and given for two months is more effective than placebo in patients with chronic low back pain.

The data analysis has to be predefined in a detailed analysis plan before the data are analyzed.

Step 1: Define the analysis population

For the primary analysis, an intention to treat analysis can be performed including all patients who were randomized and provided baseline data. As a secondary analysis, a per-protocol-analysis can be done which excludes all patients who violated the study protocol by receiving co-interventions.

Steps 2 and 3: Identify the different types of variable and clarify what you can calculate from your data

The VAS is a continuous variable and you can display means or mean changes (e.g. between baseline and two months) with SD, SE or 95 %CI. Although the back function questionnaire (HFAQ) and the quality of life questionnaire (SF-36) are categorical variables the summary scores are usually analyzed using statistics for continuous data and presenting means or mean changes. The number of days with pain medication from the diary will be analyzed as continuous data, whereas the type of drug has to be analyzed as categorical data. Safety (e.g. the number of AE and SAE) are also categorical data.

Steps 4 and 5: Choose suitable statistical procedures and perform the statistical analysis

The primary outcome is the difference in the average pain intensity (using VAS) between Devil's claw and placebo after two months of treatment. The study has one primary hypothesis: Null hypothesis: no difference between verum and placebo group in the change in the average low back pain intensity (VAS) between baseline and two months.

Alternative hypothesis: a difference between verum and placebo group in the change in the average low back pain intensity (VAS) between baseline and two months

For the primary endpoint we can use a two-sided unpaired t-test if the data are approximately normally distributed and Wilcoxon rank sum test if the data are not normally distributed. We could also apply ANCOVA adjusted for baseline values or we can discuss even more complicated models with a statistician which also control for the factor 'treatment center'.

An example of a short description of your statistical analysis could be: 'For the primary outcome (the reduction in the average pain intensity between baseline and two months on the 100 mm VAS) an ANCOVA adjusted for baseline values will be used. Missing data will be multiply imputed using regression methods.'

Step 6: Decide how you will present your results

Results can be displayed in text, tables or figures, for example: A total of 140 patients (67.8 % female; age 59 ± 9 years) were randomized (69 to Devil's claw group and 71 to placebo group). Baseline characteristics are shown in ➤ table 6.6. No significant group differences were observed at baseline.

6

Table 6.6 Baseline characteristics

	Devil's claw n = 69	Placebo n = 71	
	mean (± sd)/n (%)	mean (± sd)/n (%)	p value
Women	44 (64 %)	41 (75 %)	
Men	25 (36 %)	30 (25 %)	
Age (years)	59.1 ± 8.8	58.2 ± 9.4	0.559
Duration of LBP (years)	14.7 ± 11.0	13.6 ± 10.5	0.545
LBP intensity (VAS)	63.2 ± 13.2	66.6 ± 15.7	0.168
Back function (HFAQ)	57.1 ± 18.6	57.2 ± 17.3	0.974
Physical health (SF-36)	32.8 ± 8.2	31.8 ± 8.3	0.475
Mental health (SF-36)	48.5 ± 10.7	48.0 ± 11.1	0.787

LBP = Low Back Pain, VAS = Visual Analogue Scale, t-test for independent data

Table 6.7 Secondary outcome parameters after 2 months

	Devil's claw n = 69 mean ± sd	Placebo n = 71 mean ± sd	Difference 95 %CI	p value
Back function (HFAQ)	66.8 ± 18.3	62.9 ± 20.3	3.9 (−1.8 to 9.6)	0.235
SF-36 Physical health	40.5 ± 9.7	36.2 ± 10.3	4.3 (1.4 to 7.2)	0.012
SF-36 Mental Health	50.6 ± 9.5	51.0 ± 9.8	−0.4 (−3.2 to 2.4)	0.807

LBP = Low Back Pain, VAS = Visual Analogue Scale, t-test for independent data

6

The primary outcome, the average reduction in pain intensity after 2 months, was 28.7 ± 30.3 (mean ± sd) in the Devil's claw group compared to 23.6 ± 31.0 in the placebo group (baseline adjusted differences between groups 5.1 and 95 % CI -3.7 to 13.9, p = 0.057). Secondary outcomes are shown in ➤ table 6.7.

The per-protocol-analysis showed no relevant differences compared to the intention-to treat-analysis.

Note that this data presented here are only a short summary of the most relevant results; you will have much more data to report.

Step 7: Interpret your results and conclude

Although the p value shows a trend for Devil's claw (p = 0.057) this result is usually interpreted negatively and this should be reflected in the final conclusion. However, in the discussion a possible trend and its implications should be discussed. An example of the conclusion is: 'We found no significant difference for patients with chronic low back pain who received devils claw compared to patients who received placebo.'

Case study 3: Randomized controlled study comparing three groups

Case study 3 is a comparative effectiveness study in a usual care setting. The objective of this pragmatic, randomized three-armed trial is to evaluate whether acupuncture treatment or yoga given in addition to usual care is more effective in the treatment of patients with chronic low back pain than usual care alone and whether one of these treatments is more effective than the other. The data analysis has to be predefined in a detailed analysis plan before the data are analyzed.

Step 1: Define the analysis population

As primary analysis, an intention to treat analysis including all patients who were randomized and provided baseline data will be performed.

Steps 2 and 3: Identify the different types of variable and clarify what you can calculate from your data

Although the back function questionnaire (HFAQ) and the quality of life questionnaire (SF-36) are categorical variables the summary scores will be analyzed using statistics for continuous data. For all measures you can display means or mean changes (e.g. between baseline and three months).

Steps 4 and 5: Choose suitable statistical procedures and perform the statistical analysis

The primary outcome parameter is back function measured with the HFAQ after 3 months.

We have three primary hypotheses and two of them are tested at the same confirmatory level (acupuncture vs. usual care and yoga vs. usual care) whereas the third (yoga vs. usual care) is tested in a hierarchical order.

- Null hypothesis 1: no difference in back function between acupuncture and usual care at 3 months
- Alternative hypothesis 1: a difference in back function between acupuncture and usual care at 3 months
- Null hypothesis 2: no difference in back function between yoga and usual care at 3 months
- Alternative hypothesis 2: a difference back function between yoga and usual care at 3 months
- Null hypothesis 3: no difference in back function between acupuncture and yoga at 3 months
- Alternative hypothesis 3: a difference in back function between acupuncture and yoga at 3 months

A short summary of the statistical analysis for the primary outcome measure might be: 'To determine differences between the intervention groups and the control group after 3 months we will use ANCOVA adjusted for baseline values. Because of two primary analyses (acupuncture vs. usual care and yoga vs. usual care) Bonferroni correction will be used to address multiple testing (i.e. a significance level of 0.025 will be used). The difference between acupuncture and yoga will be tested on a confirmatory basis if both interventions differ statistically significantly from usual care (hierarchical test procedure)'.

Step 6: Decide how to present your results

A total of 600 patients (mean age 52.9 ± 13.7 years, 57.3 % female) was randomized (200 acupuncture, 200 yoga group and 200 usual care only). Baseline characteristics are shown in ➢ table 6.8.

For the primary outcome parameter of back function (HFAQ) at three months, values were 74.1 (95 % CI 73.0–75.2) in the acupuncture group, 74.6 (74.2–75.1) in the yoga group and 65.5 (64.3–66.7) in the usual care only group. A significant difference was found between acupuncture vs. usual care and yoga vs. usual care groups, $p < 0.001$ each; however, no significant difference was found between yoga and acupuncture, $p = 0.806$. The results for quality of life at 3 months are shown in ➢ table 6.9.

6

Table 6.8 Baseline characteristics

	Acupuncture n = 200	Yoga n = 200	Usual care N = 200
	mean (± SD)/n (%)	mean (± SD)/n (%)	mean (± SD)/n (%)
Women	115 (57.5 %)	119 (59.3 %)	110 (56.9 %)
Age (years)	53.1 ± 13.5	52.9 ± 13.8	52.6 ± 13.2
Duration of LBP (years)	7.2 ± 8.0	7.1 ± 7.8	7.2 ± 7.8
LBP intensity (VAS)	63.2 ± 13.2	66.6 ± 15.7	66.1 ± 13.6
Back function (HFAQ)	61.8 ± 21.0	60.6 ± 22.0	63.3 ± 20.8
Physical health (SF-36)	34.3 ± 9.0	33.8 ± 9.1	34.6 ± 9.6
Mental health (SF-36)	43.3 ± 10.3	43.5 ± 10.2	43.5 ± 10.1

LBP = Low Back Pain, VAS = Visual Analogue Scale, no significant group differences using t-test

Table 6.9 Quality of life (SF-36) changes between baseline and 3 months

	Acupuncture mean (95 % CI)	Yoga mean (95 % CI)	Usual care mean (95 % CI)	Acupuncture vs. usual care P value	Yoga vs. usual care P value
Physical health (SF-36)	7.0 (6.5;7.5)	7.9 (7.7;8.1)	2.3 (1.8;2.8)	<0.001	<0.001
Mental health (SF-36)	2.4 (1.9;2.9)	2.1 (1.9;2.4)	0.3 (-0.2;0.8)	<0.001	<0.001

Note: Beside the results displayed above, in your paper you will present further information, for example, on the follow up results at 6 and 12 months and data on safety.

Step 7: Interpret your results and conclude

For this study a conclusion could be: 'Patients with chronic low back pain, who received additional acupuncture or yoga treatment, experienced statistically significantly less pain than patients who received only usual care. No significant difference was observed between the acupuncture and the yoga groups.'

CHAPTER 7 Publication

This chapter will provide information on how to plan publication, how to write a manuscript, how to submit it for publication, and how to revise it if you receive comments from peer reviewers.

7.1 General issues

7.1.1 Why is publication so crucial?

When you finally complete your study, after years of work, it is time to make your findings available to the scientific community and, perhaps, to a wider public. Without publication your findings will remain hidden and your study will be a waste of time and resources. Not publishing your study findings is even unethical: participants agreed to undergo study procedures to increase knowledge. If you are working within a publicly funded institution, publications provide important measures of performance which often directly impact on the distribution of funding. If you apply for grants your chances will increase dramatically if you have published in respected journals.

Unfortunately, a considerable number of clinical studies remain unpublished. Major reasons for this are that studies may show ambiguous or negative results (in the sense that hypotheses or hopes were not confirmed). The lack of publication of negative or ambiguous studies is known as publication bias. It can have severe implications as the published evidence on a given topic (if summarized in a meta-analysis) might overestimate treatment effects and lead to misguided decision making.

Other reasons for not publishing are simply lack of time or lack of resources. The publication process can take a long time and sponsors are rarely willing to fund staff after the analysis is completed. If possible, try to include at least some resources for preparing a first manuscript in your budget. In many cases, however, manuscripts have to be completed or revised after a project has been completed and when you are already working on new projects.

!

To refrain from publishing findings because they are not what you wanted is scientific misconduct! But holding a nicely printed article presenting your work in your hands often gives a deep feeling of satisfaction – and you brought your project to a real end!

7.1.2 Basic things to keep in mind

There are a number of things you should keep in mind when you aim to publish successfully. Probably the most important is:

!

Write for readers, not for yourself!

Researchers who have invested a lot of effort into a study often tend to believe that the outside world is waiting to learn all the precise details of their study. But think of yourself when you have to read the work of others. We all want to see clear main messages reported in a straightforward, comprehensive, concise and understandable manner. When you write, keep imagining that you are the reader of your manuscript and think what you would like to see in this role. And keep your manuscript short! Journals typically prefer a length of 2,000 to 3,000 words (from introduction to discussion but not counting abstract, references, tables and figures).

For the majority of the world's population English is not their native language. But if you want your work to be read by the international scientific community you have to publish in English. This is not easy for many researchers, and they will often need help from native speakers checking their manuscripts.

There are some situations when it makes sense to serve your local community in your own language, but if you aim to build an international reputation this will have to be the exception.

In earlier times, books had a major role in the communication of research. These times have clearly gone for most medical research. For several decades now, all relevant original research has been published in journals. If you want your article to be read do not hide it in a book. Be aware that journals – or better their publishers and editors – have their own interests. These can be financial (making money), political (e.g. strengthening a professional society's position) or strategic (e.g. trying to outperform a higher ranking journal).

While good research should be published regardless of its results it is obvious that some news is more welcome than others. Ambiguous findings are particularly difficult to sell. Unusual news is more interesting for editors and readers than the tenth study on the same subject. But too challenging results may also be difficult to publish, particularly if you aim to get spectacular results on a highly controversial CAM method accepted in a conventional journal.

So be aware of your environment and adapt your actions accordingly during the whole process of writing the manuscript and dealing with each step of publication.

7.2 Early preparatory work

7.2.1 Define your aims

You should decide on a number of basic issues as early as possible. Who do you want to write a publication for? For specialist practitioners in your community, for conventional practitioners, for policy makers, or for a more scientifically oriented readership (most of the following sections focus on manuscripts written for this target audience)? Do you need to publish as fast as possible or are you aiming to publish in a truly prestigious journal? Do you plan to summarize your whole study in one single article or does it make sense to write several papers? In the latter case you must develop a well designed publication strategy because simultaneous submission of overlapping manuscripts is not considered acceptable by most medical journals (see http://www.icmje.org/ for more details on this issue).

7.2.2 Deciding on authorship

An important issue to decide as early as possible is a) who should be the authors of the published study and b) in what order they should appear.

Everyone who has made substantial intellectual contributions should be listed as author on the published study. According to the guidelines of the International Committee of Medical Journal Editors (ICMJE) each author listed on a publication should meet each of the following criteria:

- 1) substantial contributions to conception and design, acquisition of data, or analysis and interpretation of data;
- 2) drafting the article or revising it critically with regards to important intellectual content; and
- 3) final approval of the version to be published (www.icmje.org).

The most important but at the same time vague criterion is the first one. Ultimately the decision on authorship is a compromise between true intellectual contribution, acknowledgement of workload and political factors. As a general rule, authors on a publication should include the principal investigator and a limited number of people who have done a lot of work for the study or had important responsibilities (e.g. the statistician). If your study is small the number of authors should – as a rule of thumb – not exceed six. In a large and complex multicenter trial a larger number of authors may be necessary.

Typically, the first author of a publication has made the major intellectual contribution, for example, by conceiving the study, coordinating it and interpreting its findings. Usually, the first author is also responsible for writing the manuscript. Being the first author is the most prestigious position. However, many novices are not aware that the last author has also an important position. The last position is typically reserved for the senior author. Ideally it is the key person responsible for initiating and supervising the whole study, however, too often it is simply the head of the department or another "important" person. In principle this is not acceptable – but it is still in common practice. The first and the last positions are of major importance because they are often the only ones which count for the distribution of money and for personal careers in academic assessment processes.

Insiders know that the second author is often the person who has done most of the work (for example, the MD student who did his/her dissertation on the subject). However, this is not always the case and prestige associated with second authorship is usually no higher than with any other 'sandwich' position. If, however, the first/second position issue is difficult to resolve, it is possible to state that first and second authors contributed equally, but this solution should be exceptional. If you are not first, last or second author it matters little which position you have.

In most cases the first author is also the corresponding author responsible for all matters related to the journal regarding submission, revision and proofreading. Some journals now also request that one or more authors, referred to as "guarantors", be identified as persons who take responsibility for the integrity of the work as a whole.

Deciding on authorship can be a delicate issue and a cause of conflict. We thus strongly recommend discussing it during the planning phase. However because workload or responsibilities may change during the study, you should also discuss what circumstances may modify the order.

Functions in the publication process:

- Peer review system: all submissions which have passed editorial screening are critically evaluated by external experts
- First author: usually the principal investigator and the person who writes the manuscript
- Last author (senior author): person with an important key function in a project, often supervising the whole study
- Corresponding author: the author (most often the first or the last author) responsible for all communication with a journal (submission, revision, reprints, press contacts)
- Guarantors: persons who take responsibility for the integrity of the work as a whole
- Persons listed in the acknowledgement: "All contributors who do not meet the criteria for authorship should be listed in an Acknowledgments section. Examples of those who might be acknowledged include people who provided purely technical help or writing assistance, or the head of the department who provided only general support." (ICMJE)

7.2.3 Selecting a journal

The selection of the target journal is a crucial step in the publication process. There are thousands of medical journals, and whether your study will be read, cited, respected, discussed in the media, etc. will depend a great deal on where your article is published. This means that researchers aim to publish their manuscripts in the highest ranking journals such as the New England Journal of Medicine, JAMA, The Lancet or the British Medical Journal. However, these journals get many more manuscripts than they can publish. They can pick and choose what they consider are the best studies. All of these journals reject more than 90 % of the material they receive. So if you submit there the likelihood of having your manuscript rejected is very high. It can take less than two weeks to get your rejection (if editors consider your manuscript not interesting enough to send out for external peer review) or up to several months (if you get rejected after repeated rounds of discussion). If you repeat this process several times you lose time and you may get very frustrated. When selecting a journal you should thus consider your various interests and select the best possible compromise. The following sections give some recommendations for selecting a target journal (or a sequence of target journals).

Only submit your manuscript to a journal which is **peer-reviewed**. This is a process which means that after a first screen the editors send it out to at least two external experts who are invited to critically comment on the merits and drawbacks of the study. Peer review is clearly the best system available to ensure a) that manuscripts get improved before publication, and b) that not all nonsense gets published, but peer review is subjective and far from perfect. Journals that do not have a peer review system are usually of low scientific quality and are often guided by commercial interests.

Whenever possible, submit to a journal **listed in the database PubMed** (www.ncbi.nlm.nih.gov/pubmed). Nowadays everyone who wants to find information on a given topic in medical research almost always first searches PubMed. If you publish in a journal that is not listed it is unlikely that your article will be noticed at an international level. If you come from a country with important journals published in languages other than English you will encounter the problem that most such journals are not included in PubMed.

Although many people consider it a plague, there is little doubt that the **impact factor** is probably the most important factor for professional researchers when choosing a target journal. The impact factor is a measure of the frequency with which the "average article" in a journal has been cited in a given period of time. The impact factors of listed journals are calculated by a commercial enterprise (Thomson Institute of Scientific Information) and published yearly in the database Journal Citations Reports (JCR). At many universities JCR is accessible as part of the larger database Science Citation Index Expanded. In JCR you can search for the impact factor of single journals or you can check a group of journals. For example, you can get a list of all listed general internal medicine journals (about 100) ranked by impact factor. For 2008 the top journal – the New England Journal of Medicine – had an impact factor of 50 while the Italian journal Medicina dello Sport was at the end of the list with an impact factor of 0.1. There is also a list of "Integrative & Complementary Medicine" journals which for 2008 comprised 14 journals with impact factors between 2.8 and 0.7. If you do not have access to JCR you will find the impact factor of an individual journal on its website (if it is not reported, the journal does not have one).

The JCR database does not include a large number of journals which are listed in other databases, for example, PubMed. Due to Thomson Institute's focus on American journals, impact factors are considerably biased against European or Asian journals. The system is also self-reinforcing: high ranked journals get the best manuscripts etc. Other providers have tried to establish competing tools but up until now ISI impact factors have remained the standard and all others follow.

It is obvious that your manuscript must **fit with the subject of the target journal**. It makes little sense to submit a pragmatic clinical CAM study on back pain to a journal that mainly publishes basic pharmacological research on the neuromotor system. Once you have identified a potential target journal, screen through a number of issues to check what they typically publish and in what manner. You can also check whether the journal already published articles on topics similar to yours by searching PubMed or other databases. If your study is similar to previously published articles it can give you an advantage (the journal is open to the subject) but if there are many articles previously published in the target journal which are very similar to your study, this may turn into a disadvantage (the journal has published so much on it recently that editors and readers may be tired of seeing the same stuff again).

If possible, check the journal's editorial process for **rejection rates** and **average time from submission to decision or publication**. This will help you to consider how much time you may lose in case of rejection. From the beginning you should also look for at least one **alternative target journal** in case of rejection.

The criticism has been made that a lot of research is funded by the public only to be marketed by publishers without free access to everyone. Therefore, a large number of **open-access journals** have been established in recent years (for example, the BMC = BioMed Central journals). This has clear advantages for the author (and the readers) because articles are freely available to anyone. However, the clear drawbacks are: **publication fees**. The unavoidable costs for the whole publishing operation must now be paid by authors. You may have to pay between 1,000 and 3,000 US $ for publication fees – which is money that needs to be raised. If you consider submitting to a BMC journal, for example, check whether your institution (or the institution of a co-author) is a BMC member. If a manuscript is submitted by an author affiliated to a member institution, charges may be waived or reduced!

Criteria when selecting a journal

- Peer review system: all submissions which have passed editorial screening are critically evaluated by external experts
- PubMed listed: the journal is listed in the most important medical database
- Impact factor: the journal is included in a database (Journal Citation Reports) which checks how often an average article is cited in the literature

- Content: The subject and approach of your study fits with what is usually published in the journal
- Acceptance rate: Check what proportion of manuscripts is accepted (if websites do not provide this information the acceptance rate tends to be higher than 20 %)
- Speed: Check whether information is provided on the average time it takes from submission until a first decision is made
- Fees: Check whether you have to pay for publication

7.2.4 Checking instructions for authors

!

Once you have decided where to submit your manuscript you have to check the journal's instructions to authors carefully and of course follow them carefully.

Every professional journal has a website which provides detailed information on which articles are within its scope and what submitted manuscripts should look like. The multiplicity of instructions often entail a considerable amount of work for authors. It is impressive how creative publishers have been in devising slightly different styles. For example author names may be listed in several different ways (e.g. John Smith; Smith J; Smith J.; Smith, J.; Smith J, MD; John Smith MD, etc.). Formats for abstracts differ dramatically. And there are multiple ways of citing references. While modern referencing software (➢ Ch. 7.3.6) provides a lot of support with this, it is still good to be aware of the specific requirements of the journal as early as possible. Instructions for authors tell you how to structure your manuscript, word limits, how tables and figures should look, etc.

If you have general questions about publications, copyright issues etc. the website of the International Committee of Medical Journal Editors (ICMJE; www.icmje.org) provides valuable information.

7.2.5 Checking general guidelines for reporting

In their instructions for authors, high-ranking journals now also often require authors to follow standard recommendations for the publication of a given type of study. The most well-known example is the CONSORT guidelines for reporting randomized controlled trials. The Equator network (www.equator-network.org/home) is an international initiative of editors and scientists that lists the most relevant reporting guidelines. Following these guidelines is not only increasingly often a prerequisite for getting a study accepted but also helps authors a lot in writing.

Important reporting guidelines

- Freely accessible at www.equator-network.org/home
- Randomized controlled trials: CONSORT (www.consort-statement.org) with official extension documents for cluster trials, non-pharmacological treatments, herbal medicine trials, etc.
- Non-randomized evaluations of behavioural and public health interventions: TREND
- Systematic reviews and meta-analyses: PRISMA
- Observational studies in epidemiology: STROBE
- Diagnostic accuracy studies: STARD
- Qualitative studies: COREQ
- Reporting Interventions in Clinical Trials of Acupuncture (STRICTA)
- Not freely accessible:
- Randomized controlled trials – homeopathy: RedHot (Dean ME, Coulter MK, Fisher P, Jobst K, Walach H. Reporting data on homeopathic treatments (RedHot): a supplement to CONSORT. Homeopathy 2007;96:42–45.)
- Randomized controlled trials – Chinese herbal medicines (in Chinese): Fei YT, Liu JP. [Improving the quality of reporting Chinese herbal medicine trials: an elaborated checklist]. Zhong Xi Yi Jie He Xue Bao 2008;6:233–238.

7.3 Writing the manuscript

!

Be short and concise! Pay attention to word limits given in the instructions for authors! Do not produce too many tables and figures (in general no more than six altogether)!

Manuscripts reporting original clinical research are always structured in the same format: introduction, methods, results, discussion. But for the writing process we recommend switching the order.

7.3.1 Results section

One of us once received a very good piece of advice from a senior colleague: Always start by writing up the most important results! Summarize in a few sentences the findings for the main outcome measures.

After that you may want to proceed more systematically. Results sections of clinical studies often start by reporting the dates of the recruitment and follow-up periods, and summarizing the flow of participants through the study. If you are writing up a randomized trial, the CONSORT statement provides great guidance for doing this. Otherwise simply use good articles from high-ranking journals (or your target journal) as examples. Very often the results section is accompanied by a figure displaying a flowchart summarizing all the numbers: how many people have been approached, how many screened, how many included and excluded, how many received the interventions, how many deviated from the protocol, how many dropped out and for what reasons, how many were analyzed and how many completed the study. This figure allows the reader to get a quick overview and you do not have to give all the details in the text.

!

In general, details reported in tables or figures should not be repeated in the text.

After summarizing the patient flow, most clinical study reports describe the study participants (the study population). Again the description in the text can be rather short as all relevant detail should be given in a table which is often titled "socio-demographic characteristics and baseline values". Be careful in the selection of the characteristics for this table. In general it is probably not important to know how tall participants were and other formal details. However age, sex, possibly education, race, etc. may well be listed. In addition you should list data which allow a clinician to check whether his/her patients fit those included in the study (what were their symptoms, how long did the patients have them previous to recruitment, what medications did they take, what else did they try, what risk factors did they have). You should also include baseline values for important outcome measures, if relevant.

After these two "introduction" sections you would now insert the description of the main findings that you have started with. If you have a predefined main outcome measure and a clear hypothesis, here is the place to describe it. If possible, it is always good to have a nice figure which displays your main findings. Here you can make an exception and have both a figure and a short text description.

Then it makes sense to report the findings for the most important secondary outcomes. Typically the text is relatively short here and detailed tables and possibly some figures provide additional information.

After summarizing your main findings you may provide sensitivity analyses showing whether your results are robust (for example, if you analyze according to the per protocol instead of the intention to treat principle) or you may choose to describe subgroup analyses (for example, investigating whether providers with more or less clinical experience achieved different results).

Finally, adverse events and adverse effects should be reported in detail giving exact numbers. A summary table is often helpful.

Typical structure of a results section
- Dates of recruitment and follow up
- Flow of participants
- Findings for main outcome measure
- Findings for secondary outcome measure
- Subgroup and sensitivity analysis
- Description of adverse effects

7.3.2 Methods section

The order in the methods sections may vary slightly but very often it starts with the description of the general study design. This is often followed by the listing of the selection criteria of study participants and the methods of recruitment. The next step is typically a description of the study interventions including permitted co-interventions. When writing these descriptions you need to keep the word limit in mind but at the same time you should make the description as accurate as possible in order to allow other researchers to reproduce the study. The same applies to the reporting of outcome measurements. Clearly state which is the primary outcome measure and which are important secondary outcome measures and include the timing of the measurements. If outcome measures have been described in previous articles you do not have to go into all the details, but instead you can make reference to the earlier reports and keep your text short. If your outcome measures have been validated formally it is good to state this. The last part of a methods section typically deals with the statistics. Clearly state your formal hypothesis, describe your sample size calculation in sufficient detail, report how you handled missing values, define analysis populations, how you summarized your data descriptively and which hypothesis tests were used. For this you will probably need help from your statistician. Even if you do not have a statistician as co-author (is there a good reason for this?) you should try to have one reading your statistics section critically.

Typical structure of a methods section
- Study design
- Inclusion and exclusion criteria for study participants/recruitment
- Interventions
- Outcome measures
- Statistics (sample size calculation and analysis)

7.3.3 Introduction

Compared with articles in other disciplines such as psychology or sociology, introductory sections in medical manuscripts are short and very rarely intellectual masterpieces. They typically start with prevalence or incidence data showing that the clinical problem addressed is of utmost importance. Then the limitations of available treatments are summarized, and a statement is made that the intervention investigated is widely used/promising/controversial or important for any other reason. If there is a good rationale for the intervention studied a few phrases make sense, as well as a few words on the limitations of the evidence available so far. All this should fit onto one or two A4 pages (double-spaced) and be backed up by a few (five to ten) well-published references. Finally you should clearly state the question addressed (➢ Ch. 4.1). Use the PICO format whenever possible.

7.3.4 Discussion

Writing the discussion is usually the most challenging part – but also the most interesting. While your tone in the methods and results section must be absolutely neutral, you can enter your personal interpretation and opinion in the discussion. However, be aware that experienced editors often think that their most important task is to temper unwarranted conclusions of enthusiastic authors (Docherty & Smith 1999).

Several slightly different ways to structure discussions have been proposed to ensure that the findings of a study are put into the appropriate context. Below we have copied the proposal by Docherty & Smith (1999) for the British Medical Journal.

Proposal of Docherty and Smith (1999) for structuring discussion sections
- Statement of principal findings
- Strengths and weaknesses of the study
- Strengths and weaknesses in relation to other studies, discussing particularly any differences in results
- Meaning of the study: possible mechanisms and implications for clinicians or policymakers
- Unanswered questions and future research

The first paragraph of the discussion typically summarizes the most important findings. In the very last paragraph you briefly summarize your main conclusions and the main implications for future research and clinical practice. The contents and sequence in between is quite variable. In CAM research a discussion of mechanisms of action may often be quite speculative but if good evidence is available this can clearly increase the credibility of positive findings (if you have any). Comparing your findings with the literature is an obvious duty which may be quite difficult if your study is the first or one of the first addressing the issue. Before submitting you should have searched PubMed to make sure you have not overlooked truly relevant work. It does not cast a good light on you if you have missed the most recent relevant publications.

Inevitably, your study will have weaknesses, and if your peer reviewers are not incompetent or lazy they will put their finger exactly on the critical points. So try to figure out where the main criticism will come and try to argue in your discussion how you tried to overcome the problems or why these problems were inevitable. This is clearly a difficult job, because you want your study to be accepted and at the same time you have to show that you are able to criticize your own work. Consider asking a sceptical but open colleague to read your draft and request him to criticize you meticulously.

7.3.5 Abstract

!
The abstract of your manuscript is maybe the most important part. It is not only the first thing editors and peer reviewers will read and make their first judgement on, but it will also be the only thing the majority of readers will read.

Many journals have their own guidelines how to structure abstracts. Often they ask for a lot of detail which hardly fits into the word limit (varying typically between 150 and 250 words). In any case try to follow the structure exactly and remain within the word limit! Editors are aware that it is not always possible to include everything they ask for. The CONSORT website includes a specific document for abstracts which can be very helpful. Make sure that the content of the abstract really fits with the content of the manuscript. If possible, use the same wording as in the full text, particularly for the main findings and the conclusions. If you have to prepare an additional abstract in another language (for example, a Chinese, French or German abstract) take care that the content is identical with the English abstract.

7.3.6 References

The fact that this section is the penultimate in the writing process should not be misunderstood: when you start writing you should be very clear how you will deal with references. In the results section you do not need any references. However some references will be necessary in the methods section where you may give references for the outcome measures you use, for diagnostic classifications, etc (unless you invented everything yourself). The bulk of references will be cited in the introduction and the discussion section.

Whenever possible you should use computer software (such as Reference Manager, Endnote, ProCite) for dealing with literature. These software packages allow importing of references from major databases, storing them, cite while you write, and flexibly adapt citations to different journal formats. They all have their weaknesses and when you write your first manuscript it may make work, not save it. If you do everything by hand, be prepared that you may need to change all the numbering just before submission if you discover that you have to include a new reference.

!
Be accurate when citing and listing references.

Sloppy handling of this issue will be recognized immediately by editors and experienced reviewers and significantly decreases the credibility of your manuscript. This is a skill everyone has to master if they want to participate in the scientific ritual! And rightly so – if someone does not deal carefully with references, is it likely that they have been careful in their study?

7.3.7 Additional statements

Many journals now ask authors to declare potential conflicts of interest at the end of the manuscript and/or during the submission process. According to the World Association of Medical Editors (WAME) a "conflict of interest (COI) exists when there is a divergence between an individual's private interests (competing interests) and his or her responsibilities to scientific and publishing activities such that a reasonable observer might wonder if the individual's behavior or judgment was motivated by considerations of his or her competing interests" (www.wame.org/conflict-of-interest-in-peer-reviewed-medical-journals). Be aware that you should not only declare a conflict of interest if you have a direct financial interest in a product investigated in a study but also if, for example, you receive fees for teaching the therapy investigated in courses. Also, if you have received funding from a company who produces the product investigated, or if you have received fees or travel reimbursement, you should state this. Describing these details does not mean that your study is biased and your manuscript will be rejected – it simply means transparency. Many major conventional researchers have received funding from multiple major companies and their declarations of potential conflicts of interests are long. Nevertheless, they produce good studies which are published in high-ranking journals.

If you have received funding for your study you should also describe the source. Some journals ask that you also state whether the sponsors had any role in the design, conduct and analysis of the study, and whether they contributed to the publication. Many journals state in their instructions for authors what information they want and where it should be put. Even if they do not ask for it we recommend always describing the source of funding and the role of the sponsor. If you did not have any external funding, say so.

There may be individuals who have contributed to the study in some way but do not meet authorship criteria. For example, experienced peers may have seen early versions of the manuscript and given important comments. Laboratory technicians or administrative staff may have done a very good job. It is good practice to thank them in the acknowledgments at the end of the paper, but ask them for their consent first!

Major journals nowadays publish randomized trials only if they have been registered at the outset in trial registers (➢ Ch. 5). For other types of study this is not the case yet. If you have a trial registration number, you should include it in the manuscript (on the title page, at the end of the abstract, in the methods section or after the discussion).

7.3.8 Internal revision

A good manuscript is teamwork. If you have cooperative and competent co-authors it will be fun – even if their criticism may lead you to having to rewrite parts of your manuscript. Sometimes one author will do the first draft alone, sometimes other authors will be involved. When the first version is completed it should be circulated for comments among all authors. Give clear deadlines for their feedback. Depending on the changes recommended several feedback loops may be necessary. Not every change will need to be communicated to everyone. However, if you feel you have the "almost final" version you need to circulate this once more. Clearly instruct your co-authors that this is the last chance to suggest changes. You may consider at this stage asking your co-authors for their consent for submission. However, it is better to ask for consent with the "very final" version of the manuscript. Regardless when exactly you do it:

!

Do not submit a manuscript before each of your co-authors explicitly agreed to its content and format!

Unfortunately, it may happen that you have one or more co-authors who are not very helpful in the writing process. If possible, tell them that they may risk co-authorship if they are not doing their job. More often, however, you may have to find some way to limit their workload and just get the most basic feedback you need.

7.4 Getting your manuscript accepted

7.4.1 Preparing the submission

Finally your manuscript is completed. You carefully followed the instructions for authors. You have circulated the final version and you wait for the final consent of your co-authors. It is now time to prepare the submission.

!

Almost all scientific journals have now online submission systems.

There are a number of slightly different systems and it makes sense to explore them before actually doing the submission. Some journals have submission checklists on the authors' instruction pages but in others you will find them only on the submission page. To enable you to submit it may be necessary to register with the submission system. You will probably need an electronic submission letter where you often have to confirm that the manuscript is not simultaneously under consideration elsewhere, and that the contents have not been published. For an example of a cover letter see the box below. Sometimes instructions for authors state that you need copyright forms, but according to our experience this is rarely necessary for submission and becomes only relevant after the manuscript has been accepted. Check the instructions for authors once again point by point when you have everything ready, and read your manuscript one last time.

Example of a cover letter
Dear Dr. (*name of the editor*),
We would like to submit our manuscript
Name of the manuscript
for publication in (*name of the journal*). To the best of our knowledge this is the first study … (*Give shortly a reason why your study should be of interest to the readers of your target journal*).
The manuscript and its contents have not been published elsewhere and are not submitted elsewhere. All authors have seen and approved the final version.
We hope that you will find our manuscript interesting.
Sincerely,

7.4.2 Submitting the manuscript

When everything is ready, enter the submission site and follow the steps on the screen. If your are a novice some steps may be a bit confusing and the whole process can take up to one hour. But do not be anxious – in the end there is not a lot that can go wrong. Typically, you have to paste in the study title and the abstract, enter names, affiliations and email addresses of your co-authors, select keywords and possibly also propose potential peer reviewers. Then you will be asked to upload your manuscript files and potentially other materials.

At the end of the submission process you will be asked to check and approve the file that is constructed by the system. Then you push the "submit" button and you will be rid of it – for the moment.
Usually, you get a confirmation email including a manuscript number which is an important reference for all further communication with the journal.

7.4.3 What happens at the journal?

The details of the process depend on the journal. Very large journals have professional editors supported by teams that are sometimes large. Most speciality journals have experienced researchers as editors and a single editorial assistant or a small assisting team. But in principle the process is always the same. Each incoming manuscript is read by an editor who decides whether it merits external peer review. This should not take longer than three weeks, and if you get a decision letter that soon it is likely to be a clear rejection.

While high-ranking journals sort out the majority of submissions at that stage, most speciality journals send out the great majority of reasonable submissions to two (but up to four) external peer reviewers. To some degree peer review is a lottery. If you are lucky your manuscript ends up with someone who likes your work, but sometimes it ends up with someone who thinks it is rubbish. The main job of peer reviewers is to provide constructive criticism. Often they start their comments by giving a short overall assessment, then they describe their major concerns followed by a list of minor issues. In addition, they can give additional comments to editors which are not forwarded to authors. Some journals practise open peer review (the identity of reviewers is disclosed to the authors) but more often the reviewers remain anonymous. A number of journals do not provide authors' names and institutions to peer reviewers. Journal editors typically ask peer reviewers to provide feedback within two to four weeks. After receiving peer reviews editors should make their decision within the next two weeks. A good journal should provide you feedback with peer review within eight to ten weeks. However, the process can be prolonged by a number of issues. Some peer reviewers may not provide their feedback in time or not at all, there may be strong disagreement between peer reviewers making it necessary for editors to seek further opinions, or specific problems may be raised which have to be commented on by a specialist (e.g., statistical problems). However, if you have not received feedback after three months you should not hesitate to contact the journal.

When the review process is completed the journal sends you an email with the decision and the comments from peer reviewers. We recommend to always take a deep breath. What can you expect?

Typically journals send standard messages which include four main types of decisions:

- 1) Your manuscript is accepted straight away (without any or very minor changes) – this is very rare.
- 2) You do not get a formal acceptance yet, but the phrasing suggests that if you follow the recommendations of peer reviewers and editors you have good chances of future acceptance.
- 3) The manuscript is not accepted but you are offered to submit a revised version which can be considered again. In such cases you often get a long list of comments which may ask for considerable changes or explanations.
- 4) The manuscript is rejected definitively.

The difference between decisions 2 and 3 is fluid, and it is not always clear how long the route to acceptance is.

7.4.4 Revision

If the decision letter asks you to submit a revised version of your manuscript take another deep breath before reading the comments from peer reviewers. The comments are likely to include things you will not like at all, some will exactly hit the critical issues but you may perceive some as completely stupid. If you are lucky, you will receive recommendations which are easy to follow and will improve your manuscript. In most cases, however, it won't be that easy. Forward the decision letter to all of your co-authors as well. If you are emotional we suggest that you sleep over the whole issue at least once.

In general we would recommend the following approach for dealing with the comments:

!

In a response letter answer each single point raised by peer reviewers and editors in a cooperative and clear manner.

It is usually entirely acceptable not to follow all recommendations if you explain why. However, you should not reject every comment. Try to follow the recommendations where it makes some sense. Some journals ask that you provide a version where the changes are marked.

If you have completed a draft of the response letter and of the revised manuscript circulate it among all authors. If the revision is minor it may be sufficient to simply inform your co-authors, but if major changes are necessary they should approve a new final version explicitly. Before resubmitting check once again whether you have addressed all relevant issues and whether the tone of your replies is truly appropriate. Avoid arguments.

The BMC (Biomed Central) journals publish the "pre-publication history" of each manuscript on their websites. This is a very good way to learn what peer review looks like and how response letters may be written.

If you are lucky you will soon receive a letter telling you that your manuscript is now accepted or will be accepted if you do this or that further small formal change. This is usually a very satisfying moment. If you are less lucky you wait several weeks and the whole game is repeated – sometimes with, sometimes without a happy ending.

7.4.5 After rejection …

It is a normal part of every researcher's life to get manuscripts rejected. It is not unusual to have a manuscript rejected two or three times, and sometimes it happens even more often. This can be time consuming and very frustrating. Try to consider rationally what the problems have been and how to increase the chances of getting the manuscript accepted. This may mean that you modify your manuscript, that you try a lower ranking journal, that you choose a journal in another discipline or in another part of the world, etc. In each case make sure when resubmitting that you followed the author guidelines of the new journal. If editors see from the format that your manuscript was clearly written for another journal it is unlikely to increase their sympathy level. In any case, do not give up too early. Most manuscripts get accepted sooner or later …

7.5 After acceptance

7.5.1 Proofreading

In most cases you get your manuscript accepted eventually. You will probably have to fill in some forms and provide signatures for copyright, authorship and regarding conflicts of interests. It will then takes some weeks or months until you, if you are the corresponding author, receive the page proofs of your manuscript. You will then be asked to send the corrected proofs back very fast: typically within 72 hours. Be really careful when reading the proofs.

!

> Proofreading is the last chance to correct errors you have made yourself or those that have been introduced during the production of the typescript.

You are not allowed to make major text changes (publishers will charge you if they need to redo the production due to some new foolish idea of yours). Particularly, check figures and tables as these are often newly produced for printing. Also check that citations and references are correct as these are often produced automatically.

7.5.2 Finally: Publication

Sooner or (mostly) later the big moment comes. Your manuscript is published. Nowadays most articles are published initially in an electronic format online because the printing process takes additional time. Electronic publications can be cited without any problem. They have a unique identification number (so-called doi). They look like the final print but the final page numbers relating to the printed journal issue are missing. Many journals provide you with a pdf version for limited circulation but sometimes you have to pay for your own article.

7.5.3 Dealing with mass media

Most often nobody cares about your article outside a limited research community. But occasionally you may be contacted by the press, radio or television. If you are contacted before publication you should not disclose any information. Large journals provide advance information shortly before publication to accredited media representatives. Editors will inform you in that case and tell you what you have to do.

When speaking to the press make sure that you see a draft of the article before publication for a check. Be aware that information in the mass media must always be short, simple – and most of all – interesting to readers. This can result in quite biased representation of your work if you do not take care. But fortunately, quite a number of journalists do a great job. And let's be honest – who does not feel flattered to read their name in a big newspaper or see their face on TV?

REFERENCE

Docherty M, Smith R. The case for structuring the discussion of scientific papers. BMJ 1999;318:1,224–5.

FURTHER READING

Browner WS. Publishing and presenting clinical research. Second edition. Philadelphia: Lippincott, Williams & Wilkins, 2006.

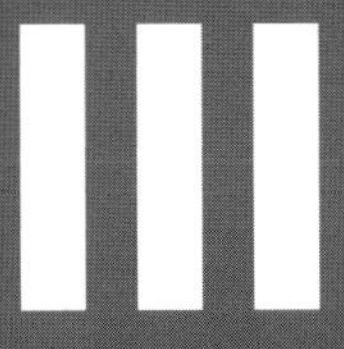

Putting a clinical study into context

Part 3 of the book contains an introduction to methods relevant to putting the findings of efficacy and effectiveness studies into a broader context. Chapter 8 deals with qualitative research which can provide relevant insights into beliefs, attitudes, motivation, processes, and perceived changes that go beyond numbers. Chapter 9 summarizes the basics of health economics, a field of increasing importance in time of limited resources. Since individual cases are at the very heart of every health care profession, we give an overview, in chapter 10, on the use of single-case research methods to evaluate complementary therapies. Finally, in chapter 11, we shortly introduce other important study designs (studies on diagnosis, etiology and prognosis, and cross-sectional studies) in clinical and epidemiological research not covered in detail in this book.

CHAPTER

8 Qualitative research

Qualitative health research seeks out to understand the 'what', 'how' or 'why' of a phenomenon. It doesn't rely on statistics or numbers, instead it works with texts, pictures, and videos. Research questions arise from particular theoretical frameworks and qualitative research is used to gain insight into people's attitudes, behaviors, value systems, concerns, motivations, aspirations, culture or lifestyles. Qualitative research does not seek to prove or disprove hypotheses; it aims to explore situations, interactions, and the lives of people without judgment. As with all research it is crucial to think about what you want to investigate and then make sure that qualitative methods are the right methodology for your research question. Qualitative research has a vast and complex area of methodology and we can only provide a very short overview. Within this book qualitative research is presented as a method which can be useful to inform quantitative research. Quantitative research is more often confirmatory and deductive in nature, whereas qualitative research in the health field is used in an exploratory and inductive manner. The purpose of this section is to introduce you to the idea of qualitative research (and how it is related to quantitative research) and to give you some orientation to the major types of qualitative research tools, approaches and methods. If you want to do qualitative research you should find an experienced qualitative researcher for supervision of your project.

A combination of both qualitative and quantitative research could be beneficial. For example, you have planned a RCT which compares Yoga with physiotherapy for patients with chronic neck pain. In addition you would like to gather information about patients' expectations, about patients' treatment response and believe systems behind the expectation. You then have to decide about the type of interview, how you select the patients to be interviewed and how you analyze their answers. For this you will need advice of an experienced qualitative researcher.

It is important to be aware that qualitative research produces large amounts of textual data in the form of transcripts and observational field notes. The systematic and rigorous preparation and analysis of these data is time consuming. High quality analysis of qualitative data depends on the skill, vision, and integrity of the researcher; it should not be left to the novice.

8.1 Research question and examples

Just like quantitative research, in qualitative research the first step is to identify the research questions. The theoretical framework helps shape the kind of questions asked in qualitative research. The design then depends on the kinds of questions and methodological preferences. If you need answers to questions such as 'How many patients use acupuncture for back pain?' a quantitative design is more appropriate. If you want to understand the perspective of the patient, for example, 'Why is he or she using acupuncture for back pain?' the qualitative approach allows a deeper understanding. It may be necessary to combine different qualitative methods to answer a question, for example, observation and interviews. Sometimes it is not feasible to use the most appropriate methodology to answer your research question, for example, if you are interested in a very private behavior, such as sexual behavior you might be restricted to interviews rather than direct observation. In addition sometimes the most appropriate method, for example observation, may not be used because there is not enough time or not enough financial backing for this resource-intense research setting. Framing the research question and developing the adequate research design depends on both the theoretical framework and external factors such as feasibility and funding.

Examples of qualitative research studies are shown below (➤ examples 1 and 2):

EXAMPLE 1

Hughes JG, Goldbart J, Fairhurst E, Knowles K. Exploring acupuncturists' perceptions of treating patients with rheumatoid arthritis. Complement Ther Med. 2007 Jun;15(2):101–8.

Aims: To outline acupuncturists' perceptions of treating patients with rheumatoid arthritis, exploring the impact of practitioner affiliation to a traditional or western theoretical base.

Methods: Qualitative study utilising Grounded Theory Method. Nineteen acupuncturists were chosen via theoretical sampling. In-depth semi-structured interviews were tape-recorded and transcribed. Field notes were also taken. Emerging categories and themes were identified.

Results: Inter-affiliatory differences were identified in the treatments administered and the scope and emphasis of intended therapeutic effects. Limited divergence was found between acupuncturists' perceptions of treatment outcomes. Factors perceived as impacting on treatment outcomes were identified.

Conclusions: Clinical trials of acupuncture in rheumatoid arthritis may have failed to administer a treatment which reflects that administered in clinical practice. Outcome measures employed in clinical trials of acupuncture in rheumatoid arthritis, as well as established outcome indices for rheumatoid arthritis, may lack the necessary breadth to accurately assess acupuncture's efficacy. Acupuncturist affiliation has demonstrable implications for the practice and research of acupuncture.

EXAMPLE 2

Pawluch D, Cain R, Gillett J. Lay constructions of HIV and complementary therapy use. Soc Sci Med. 2000 Jul;51(2):251–64.

This study examines the meanings that individuals with HIV attach to their use of complementary therapies. A qualitative analysis of 66 interviews completed between 1993 and 1998 showed that complementary therapies represent different things for these individuals: a health maintenance strategy, a healing strategy, an alternative to Western medicine, a way of mitigating the side-effects of drug therapies, a strategy for maximizing quality of life, a coping strategy, and a form of political resistance. We found that the meanings individuals ascribe to complementary therapies and the benefits they expect to derive from them are not idiosyncratic, but linked to social characteristics, sexuality, ethnocultural background, gender and to beliefs about health and illness, values and experiences. We found as well that these meanings are neither mutually exclusive nor exceed. The therapies often appeal to individuals on different levels and their appeal may change over time.

8.2 Qualitative approaches

Qualitative research is used in many disciplines, for example social science, anthropology and psychology. Examples for qualitative approaches are ethnography, field research, and case studies.

8.2.1 Ethnography

The ethnographic approach comes mainly from the field of anthropology and emphasizes to study an entire culture. Originally, the idea of a culture was tied to the notion of ethnicity and geographic location, but it has been broadened to include virtually any group or organization, such as the 'culture' of a traditional treatment (e.g. Chinese Medicine). Ethnography is an extremely broad area with a great variety of methods including quantitative assessment. The most basic ethnographic approach is participant observation as part of field research. The researcher becomes an active participant of the "culture" and records extensive observations. There is no preset limit of what will be observed and no real end point in an ethnographic study.

8.2.2 Field research

The essential idea of field research is that the researcher goes 'into the field' to observe the phenomenon in its natural state, for example, by working in a hospital for Chinese medicine for several weeks. As such, it is probably most related to the method of participant observation. The field researcher typically takes extensive field notes which are subsequently coded and analyzed in a variety of ways.

8.2.3 Case studies

A case study is an intensive study of a specific individual or specific context, for example, the acupuncture service as part of the Integrative Medicine Service at the Memorial Sloan-Kettering Cancer Center. It could also be a case study of several individuals using CAM for a specific condition. There is no single way to conduct a case study, and a combination of methods (e.g. interviews or direct observation) can be used.

8.3 Qualitative methods and types of data

There are a wide variety of methods that are commonly used as qualitative measurement. In fact, the methods are largely limited by the imagination of the researcher. Here we show a few of them and the different types of data. Qualitative data include any information that can be captured and are not numerical in nature.

8.3.1 Interviews

This includes both individual interviews and interviews with groups (e.g. focus groups). The data can be recorded in different ways including stenography, audio recording, video recording or written notes. Audio recording is very often used. In interviews there is a researcher who asks the questions and one or more interviewees. The purpose of the interview is to probe the ideas of the interviewees on the subject of interest. There are two main types: **unstructured interviews** and **semi-structured interviews**. Both involve direct interaction between the researcher and one interviewee or a group of them. Unstructured interviewing differs from semi-structured interviews in two main aspects: although the researcher may have a brief topic guide or core concepts to ask about, there is no formal structured or semi-structured interview guide and the interviewer is free to move the conversation in any direction of interest that may come up. The interview takes more the form of a conversation than a question answer session. Consequently, unstructured interviewing is particularly useful for exploring a topic broadly. However, there is a price for this lack of structure. Because each interview tends to be unique with no predetermined set of questions asked of all respondents, it is usually more difficult to analyze unstructured interview data, especially when synthesizing across interviewees. For semi-structured interviews the researcher has an interview guide with a list of themes and potential questions. The interview style still has flexibility allowing an open dialogue that can extend the list of topics on the interview guide. The advantage of the semi-structured approach is that similar topics are addressed in all interviews. In health research most interviews are recorded and afterwards transcribed. Written text can be more easily organized and coded than audio tapes.

8.3.2 Observation

Direct observation differs from interviewing in that the observer does not formally query the observed. It can include everything from field research where one lives in another context or culture for a period of time to photographs that illustrate some aspect of the subject matter. The data can be recorded in many of the same ways as interviews (stenography, audio, video) and through photos (e.g. photos of the practice setting).

Participant observation

One of the most common methods for qualitative data collection, participant observation is also one of the most demanding. It requires that the researcher becomes a participant in the culture or context being observed. The literature on participant observation discusses the role of the researcher as a participant, the collection and storage of field notes, and the analysis of field data. Participant observation often requires months or years of intensive work as its goal is a thorough understanding of the entire complex phenomenon under study.

Direct observation

Direct observation differs from participant observation in a number of ways. Firstly, a direct observer doesn't typically become a participant in the context. However, the direct observer does strive to be as unobtrusive as possible so as not to bias the observations. Secondly, direct observation suggests a more detached perspective. The researcher is watching rather than taking part. Consequently, technology can be a useful part of direct observation. For instance, one can videotape the phenomenon or observe from behind one-way mirrors. Thirdly, direct observation tends to be more focused than participant observation. The researcher is observing certain sampled situations or people rather than trying to become immersed in the entire context. Finally, direct observation tends not to take as long as participant observation. For instance, one might observe child-mother interactions under specific circumstances in a laboratory setting from behind a one-way mirror, looking especially for the nonverbal cues that are used.

8.3.3 Written documents or pictures

Qualitative research can also use written documents or pictures. These may include articles in newspapers or magazines, books, websites, movies, memos, transcripts of conversations, annual reports, and even patients' drawings, e.g. as part of art therapy.

8.4 Qualitative data analysis

Qualitative data analysis is a complex process and the necessary skills are difficult to develop. It comes from high quality social science training and from long term experience. There is no 'recipe book' how to do this analysis and the analysis already starts during the data collection, which allows the researcher to go back, refine questions and to develop hypotheses.

On a practical level the data are initially approached by reading several times through the notes or transcripts and writing notes and discussing the forthcoming ideas with colleagues. Within the process the data are broken down and categorized to allow the identification of concepts, however, it is also important to detect and document atypical cases, conflicts and contradictions in the data. There are two main approaches to analyzing the data.

8.4.1 Content analysis

Content analysis is a widely used qualitative research technique. Rather than being a single method, there are several approaches and all of them are used to interpret meaning from the content of text data. With a directed approach, content analysis starts with a theory or relevant research finding as guidance for initial codes and uses a kind of 'recipe book' from the beginning. When themes appear in the data codes are used to label these sentences or paragraphs. However, during the process of data analysis further codes may be developed. During the analysis process the different stages of the results are documented in notes.

8.4.2 Grounded theory

Grounded theory is a research method in which the theory is developed from the data, rather than the other way round. That makes it an inductive approach which means that it moves from the specific to the more general. The basic idea of the grounded theory approach is to read the data, e.g. memos from participant observation on the transcript of an interview and discover categories or concepts and their interrelationships. Initially open coding is used. Open coding is the part of the analysis concerned with identifying, naming, categorizing and describing phenomena found in the text. Essentially, each line, sentence, paragraph etc. is read in search of the answer to the repeated question 'What is this about? What is being referenced here?' The labels refer to things like case taking, patient-practitioner-interaction, relaxation, etc. They are the nouns and verbs of a conceptual world. Part of the analytical process is to identify the more general categories the data fall into. We also seek out the adjectives and adverbs for the properties of these categories. It is important to have fairly abstract categories in addition to very concrete ones, as the abstract ones help to generate general theory. Later, one moves to more selective coding where one systematically codes with respect to a core concept. Initially the data are read and re-read to identify and index themes and categories: these may center on particular phrases, incidents, or types of behavior. The codes and categories evolve from data as an ongoing process, however, the analysis of each interview has to be started again, screening for the new developed categories until no more new information appears. In addition the theories arising in the beginning may be checked in the later material.

Recording the thoughts and ideas of the researcher as they evolve throughout the study is done by using memos. Early in the process these memos tend to be very open while later on they tend to increasingly focus in on the core concept. Diagrams are used to pull all of the detail together, to help make sense of the data with respect to the emerging theory. The diagrams can be any form of graphic that is useful at that point in theory development or in the form of a mind map. This work is best done in group sessions where different members of the research team are able to interact and share ideas to increase insight.

8.5 Quality assurance in qualitative research

Compared to quantitative research qualitative research seems to be very subjective, because observations, interviews and the data analysis can be strongly influenced by each researcher. Qualitative researchers are aware of this limitation and record the self-observed behavior and feelings during data collection and data analyzes in memos. These notes are part of the material which is reflected in the data analyses and interpretation of the results. In addition it is important to work in a team and to discuss the results: A qualitative researcher must not work alone!

Working in a research group could be used to increase the validity of data analyses and data interpretation and is essential for those working with grounded theory. For example the coding could be done by more than one researcher and group discussions could be used during data analyzes and interpretation. Nevertheless, for the quality of qualitative research the experience and knowledge of the researcher plays a tremendous role and junior researchers should find a qualified supervisor.

Collecting and analyzing this unstructured information can be messy and time-consuming when using only manual methods. When faced with bigger volumes of material computers are useful for administrative functions, for example, arranging and sorting data. However, what computers cannot do is think like a qualitative researcher. There is a variety of software available which is specialized on qualitative research (e.g. Atlas-ti and MaxQdata)

8.6 Combining qualitative and quantitative research methods

Mixed-Method-Research is a synonym for the combination of qualitative and quantitative methods within a research project (➤ example 3).

EXAMPLE 3

MacPherson H, Thorpe L, Thomas K. Beyond needling – therapeutic processes in acupuncture care: a qualitative study nested within a low-back pain trial. J Altern Complement Med. 2006 Nov;12(9):873–80.

Background: In the medical and scientific literature, there is a dearth of reports about how acupuncturists work and deliver care in practice. An informed characterization of the treatment process is needed to support the appropriate design of evaluative studies in acupuncture.

Methods: The design was that of a nested qualitative study within a pragmatic clinical trial. Six acupuncturists who treated up to 25 patients each were interviewed after the treatment phase of the trial to obtain an account of their experiences of providing acupuncture care to patients with low back pain referred by their GP. Using semistructured interviews and a topic guide, data were collected and analyzed for both a priori and emergent themes. This paper focuses on practitioners' accounts of the goals and processes of care, and describes the strategies employed in addition to needling and other hands-on treatments.

8

Results: From the interview data, it is clear that a coherent body of theoretical knowledge informed clinical decisions and practice, and that the goals of treatment went beyond the alleviation of immediate pain-related symptoms. Acupuncturists in this study all described a pattern of patient-centered care based on a therapeutic partnership. Study participants confirmed the importance of three processes that characterized acupuncture care in this trial, each contributing to the goal of a positive long-term outcome; building a therapeutic relationship; individualizing care; and facilitating the active engagement of patients in their own recovery. Acupuncturists described elements of care that characterized these processes including establishing rapport, facilitating communication throughout the period of care, using an interactive diagnostic process, matching treatment to the individual patient, and the use of explanatory models from Chinese medicine to aid the development of a shared understanding of the patient's condition and to motivate lifestyle changes that reinforce the potential for a recovery of health. Acupuncturists did not view these therapeutic goals, processes, and strategies as a departure from their usual practice.

Conclusions: This study suggests that acupuncture care for patients with chronic conditions such as low back pain is likely to be a complex intervention that utilizes a number of patient-centered strategies to elicit longterm therapeutic benefits. Research designed to evaluate the effectiveness of acupuncture as it is practiced in the UK needs to accommodate the full range of therapeutic goals and related treatment processes.

It can answer a broader and more complete range of research questions because the researcher is not confined to a single method or approach. The use of the mixed-method approach is likely to increase the quality of final results and to provide a more comprehensive understanding of analyzed phenomena. Mixed methods research offers great promise for practicing researchers who would like to see methodologists describe and develop techniques that are closer to what practitioners actually do in practice. However, it can be difficult for a single researcher to carry out both qualitative and quantitative research; it may require a research team and an openness towards other theoretical and methodological approaches by all involved.

FURTHER READING

Judith Green & Nicky Thorogood Qualitative Methods for Health Research. 2nd Edition Sage Publications London, 2009.

Steiner Kvale: InterViews: An Introduction to Qualitative Research Interviewing. Sage Publications London, 1996.

CHAPTER

9 Economic studies

Decision makers are increasingly faced with the challenge of reconciling growing demand for health care services with available funds (Williams 1988). Assessing the impact of investments in research to prevent, detect, and treat diseases answers questions such as whether consumers are getting good value for the money spent. The underlying assumptions of economics is that the resources available to the society as a whole are scarce and decisions have to be made about their best use. This is true for health care as well as for any other resource area. Nevertheless, dealing with results from health economic evaluations is an ethical issue, because there is an implication that some patients will be refused or not offered treatment for the sake of other patients and, yet such choices have been made and are being made all the time.

Although there are multiple uses for cost estimates in health care research and policy making, the majority of applications fall into two broad categories (Lipscomb et al. 2009):

1. Assessments of the aggregate economic burden of disease and illness

This is typically done at the population level, e.g., the net cost impact in the United States of cardiovascular disease in 2009, or that the total global burden of disease resulting from neuropsychiatric disorders is projected to rise to 14.7 % by 2020. Such burden-of-illness studies may focus not only on the overall burden of specific diseases or disease groups, but also on the cost implications of health behaviors (e.g. smoking) and health conditions (e.g. obesity) that have multiple health consequences. Burden-of-illness studies may also assess population level interventions to impact costs and health outcomes by influencing behaviors (e.g. cigarette excise taxes) or reducing population disease and illness rates.

2. Economic evaluations of specific health care interventions or programs

These could be, for example, the assessment of cost-effectiveness for a new drug or a complex rehabilitation method. Such evaluations may also include cost-benefit and cost-identification analyses, as well as budget impact analyses to assess the financial impact and feasibility of interventions.

The following chapter will give an overview about the basic principles and types of economic analyses. In addition, it will give some guidance on the critical appraisal and some examples for cost-effectiveness evaluations on CAM. If you plan to include an economic evaluation into your study you should contact a health economist for advice.

9.1 Principles of economic analysis

9.1.1 Costing

Categorization of costs

Costs could be divided into direct, indirect and intangible costs. **Direct costs** include those resources directly arising from the provision of health care, such as the time spent by health care professionals (and those from other agencies such as social services), medicines, equipment and patients' costs to receive treatment (e.g. traveling time and expenses). **Indirect costs** – also known as costs due to reduced human productivity – represent the impact of illness and treatment on paid and non-paid work time (and the ability to work) and on leisure time. **Intangible costs** take into account the pain and suffering that result from undergoing a treatment. They are very rarely included in economic evaluations, but may be captured on the outcome side in part by quality of life measures.

Perspective of the study

The perspective of the study determines the included cost components. The perspective is the point of view from which the economic analysis is undertaken. The **societal perspective** is the most comprehensive approach and includes all costs and effects that are relevant as seen from the viewpoint of society, including indirect costs caused by the disease under investigation, such as production loss. The **patient perspective** includes all costs that are relevant from the viewpoint of the patient. The **health services perspective** (frequently mentioned as third party payer's perspective) is mostly used to provide economic information to decision makers. It is distinct from the societal perspective in that it takes into account only the cost of the provision of the health service. In an analysis conducted from the health services perspective some direct and indirect costs are excluded, for example, the patients' travel costs or costs arising from production loss.

Overall cost analysis and disease specific cost analysis

A cost analysis may be **disease-specific** only or it may have a wider focus and include all cost data (**overall costs**) for a patient independent of the diagnosis of interest. For a disease-specific cost analysis, all costs that are directly associated with the disease under study have to be identified.

Discounting

If a study is longer than 12 months the costs and effects have to be discounted. Discounting is a technique which allows the calculation of the present value of future costs or future effects of healthcare interventions. Discounting of health effects is based on time preference which assumes that individuals prefer to have a small part of the effects immediately, rather than to receive the full effects only in the (uncertain) future. The concept assumes that individuals prefer to delay costs rather than to incur them in the present, because the expected economic growth will give them more money in the future. The discounting rate, which is used in economic evaluations to discount the future health gains and future costs, varies for each country. The guidelines for economic evaluation usually recommend an equal discounting rate for costs and effects and the WHO recommends a global discounting rate of 3 % for both costs and effects, but a variation of this rate in sensitivity analysis, within a realistic range, is essential.

Limitations

One major source of difficulty lies with the data, because in most cost analyses, the data on which cost data is based were created for purposes other than health care costing (e.g. reimbursement). For various reasons, the posted prices of health care goods and services often do not convey accurate or useful information about economic costs. The health care system produces literally thousands of heterogeneous products, whose individual prices are often not observed in the complex maze of pricing for bundled services. Moreover, observed prices may reflect differences in market power between buyers and sellers (as reflected, for example, in negotiated price discounts), efforts to cross-subsidize unprofitable services, and other market imperfections and idiosyncrasies (Lipscomb et al. 2009).

9.1.2 Measuring the benefit

Outcomes from treatments and other health-influencing activities have two basic components – the quantity and the quality of life. Life expectancy is a traditional measure (e.g. still often used in cancer studies) with few problems for comparison – people are either alive or not. However, overall a broad range of outcome measures exists and they may be objective, subjective or patient centered (➤ Ch. 4.8). Measuring outcomes is complex, although one treatment may help someone to live longer, it may also have serious side effects. For example, it may make them feel sick, put them at risk of other illnesses or leave them permanently disabled. Another treatment may not help someone to live as long, but it may improve their quality of life while they are alive, for example, by reducing their pain or disability (e.g. palliative care). An attempt to measure and value quality of life is a more recent innovation, with a number of approaches being used (➢ Ch. 4.8). **The Quality Adjusted Life Year (QALY)** method helps us measure these factors. www.nice.org.uk/newsroom/features/measuringeffectivenessandcost-effectivenesstheqaly.jsp (January 2010) In addition, these approaches can help to compare the results from different treatments for the same or different conditions. However, it is of note that comparisons between different diagnoses are problematic and in some countries are not accepted, e.g. Germany.

Quality Adjusted Life Years (QALY)

The QALY is a measure of disease burden and combines both the quality and the quantity of life. A QALY gives an idea of how many extra months or years of life of a reasonable quality a person might gain as a result of treatment. This is particularly important when considering treatments for chronic conditions. The quality of life is represented by using **utility values (utilities)** (➢ Fig. 9.1).

If the extra years would not be lived in full health, for example if the patient would lose a limb, or be blind, then the extra life-years are valued between 0 and 1 to account for this (e.g. 0.4).

The QALY is the product of a utility value, which represents the quality of live and the quantity of life in years. The following box gives an example for the calculation of a QALY.

There is a group of patients with breast cancer. If they continue to receive standard treatment they will live on average for 1 year and their quality of life will be 0.4 (0 or below = worst possible health, 1 = best possible health)
If they receive, in addition to the standard treatment, a complex CAM intervention they will live for 1 year 3 months (1.25 years), with a quality of life of 0.5.
Standard treatment: 1 (year's extra life) × 0.4 = 0.4 QALY
Standard treatment plus additional treatment: 1.25 year (this means 3 months extra life) × 0.5 = 0.625 QALYs
Therefore, the additional treatment leads to 0.225 additional QALYs (0.625–0.4 QALY = 0.225 QALYs).

QALYs have been used in the assessment of health interventions for three decades. The popularity of the QALY approach has been constantly increasing, although the debate on its theoretical underpinnings and practical implications is still ongoing (Sassi 2006).

Determining the utility values

There are some accepted methods for developing utilities such as the time trade-off method, the standard gamble or simple rating scales. All of them have disadvantages which include that they are time consuming and that high qualified interviewers are needed. Their validity depends on the sample of respondents and there is still an ongoing discussion how this sample should be chosen (i.e. from the public, from health professional or from patients). Another option is to use health related quality of life measures to calculate utilities. Here the most common methods will be introduced.

Time trade-off method

This method involves asking respondents to establish equivalence. Respondents are asked to consider an illness that is to last for a fixed period of time. They are informed that a new treatment will give back the normal health for a shorter period of time, but with the likelihood of death or severe disablement at the end of that time. The time spent in normal health is varied until the respondent is unable to make a choice of one option.

For example the respondents have the choice to either live with lung cancer under chemotherapy for 'x' years or to live 't' years in perfect health. By

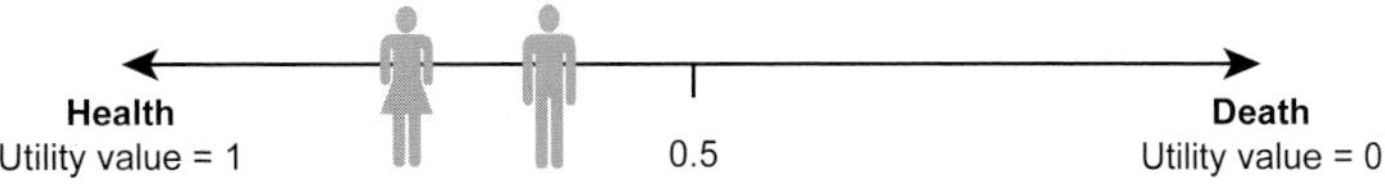

Fig. 9.1 Utility values: each period of time in perfect health is assigned the value of 1.0 down to a value of 0.0 for death

9

varying 'x', the amount of time at which the respondent is indifferent is determined. The ratio 'x/t' quantifies the preference for the specific state of health. If 1 year in perfect health was considered as valuable as 3 years with chemotherapy the utility value is ⅓ = 0.33.

The standard gamble method

This method asks the respondent to make a choice between either remaining in a current state of illness or the possibility of being immediately restored to perfect health with some risk of immediate death.

For example the respondents have the choice to either continue living in the current state of health (e.g., lung cancer), or to let chance decide on their health status. They have the chance to be healed with a probability 'p' and the chance to die with a probability '1–p'. 'P' is varied until the participant is unable to make a choice. As a result, 'p' represents the utility of the current state of health.

Rating scale method

It is also possible to determine utility values with a visual analog scale (VAS), where at one end '0' is equal to being dead and at the other end '100' is equal to being in full health. This scale is given to patients in a study with a certain state of disease. For example, if osteoarthritis of the knee with a Kellgren grade 3 is judged to be 75 mm (= 0.75 as utility value), then the patient perceived this state to reduce his or her health status by a quarter.

Health-related quality of life measures

Health-related quality of life measures are often used to determine QALYs in clinical studies.

Two standardized measures for health-related quality of life which could be used to calculate utility values are the 36-item Short Form Health Survey (SF-36) (Ware & Sherbourne 1992) and the Euroquol EQ 5D (www.euroqol.org). In addition, the shorter version of the SF-36, the SF-12, may be used to calculate QALYs. You will find published routines on how to calculate utilities from these surveys in the relevant literature.

9.2 Types of economic evaluations

There are three main types of economic analyses: cost of disease analysis, cost-benefit analysis and cost-effectiveness analysis. Cost-utility and cost-minimization analyses are subcategories of the cost-effectiveness analysis (➤ Table 9.1). The main difference between the types of economic evaluations is the measure of benefits.

9.2.1 Cost of disease analysis

The cost of disease analysis takes only costs into account without any regard to outcome. This analysis is often used by health insurances or national health systems to identify the burden of diseases and to allocate health care resources. The following box gives an example of a cost of disease analysis.

Example

In patients with migraine the average cost in the year 2010 was 3,120 € with a standard deviation of 2,785 €, according to their health insurance company.

Table 9.1 Types of economic analyses

Analyses type	Costs	Benefit	Characteristics
Cost-of-disease or burden of illness	monetary	-	Cost analysis only
Cost-benefit	monetary	monetary	Benefit measured monetary
Cost-effectiveness	monetary	naturalistic	Effectiveness differs
Cost-utility	monetary	naturalistic (e.g., QALYs)	Utility differs
Cost-minimization	monetary	naturalistic (e.g. lives saved)	Equal effectiveness

9.2.2 Cost-benefit analysis

A cost-benefit analysis refers to approaches that assign a monetary value to the benefits of an intervention and compare this with the monetary cost of the intervention. It is of note that both sides (costs and outcome) are monetary measures. The advantage is that there is a clear measure without the worry about different and complex outcome measures. However, it is difficult to express health outcomes only as costs (e.g. saved hospital days in Euros) and since this is a hotly debated ethical issue, the concept of cost-benefit analysis is not often used in medicine.

9.2.3 Cost-effectiveness-analysis

The cost-effectiveness analysis assesses efficiency i.e. the measurement of outcomes in 'natural units' (e.g. mmHg of systolic blood pressure, or mm on pain VAS) and compares these with the monetary costs of the health care given.

!

If a therapeutic intervention is both, more effective but also more expensive compared to a reference option, an incremental cost-effectiveness-analysis should be performed.

The incremental cost-effectiveness of a health care intervention is defined as the ratio of net change in health care costs to net change in health outcomes. Whether the more costly intervention is cost-effective will however depend on the willingness to pay for one additional outcome unit. If the additional cost for one additional outcome unit is lower than the willingness to pay, the treatment under consideration should be cost-effective, even though it is more expensive than the comparative treatment.

The following box will give an example.

Example

A study compares the effectiveness of a standard drug treatment with acupuncture for patients with low back pain.
After 3 months of drug treatment only, the pain measured on a pain scale is reduced on average by 13 mm, whereas in the acupuncture group a reduction of 23 mm was observed.
Costs for the standard drug treatment were 50 € and for the acupuncture treatment 350 €.
The additional cost was thus 300 € in the acupuncture group and this resulted in 10 mm additional pain reduction, or in other words and extra 30 € were spent for each mm of pain reduction achieved by the acupuncture treatment. If the willingness to pay for one mm lower pain is higher than 30 €, the acupuncture can be considered as a cost-effective treatment.

If the outcome measure is mortality the results of different studies may be comparable, however, other outcome measures especially for chronic diseases vary greatly which makes any comparison of the results of cost-effectiveness analyses between studies nearly impossible. Cost effectiveness-analyses have further limits, since they cope badly with more than one outcome. For example, if a new cancer treatment results in longer life expectancy than the existing one, but has more side effects, only one of the two outcomes can be used for the cost-effectiveness analysis (usually the life expectancy). The result will thus only represent part of the whole outcome. However, this is not primarily a problem of economic analysis because it occurs also in clinical studies where often only one primary endpoint is defined. A method to account for the benefits and side effects and to allow a better comparison of the results between studies in economic studies is the so called cost-utility analysis.

Incremental Cost Effectiveness Ratio

The Incremental Cost Effectiveness Ratio (ICER) is defined as the ratio of the difference in the cost of a therapeutic intervention, compared to the alternative intervention, to the difference in the effects of the two interventions.

$$ICER = \frac{\text{Difference in cost (intervention 1} - \text{intervention 2)}}{\text{Difference in outcome (intervention 1} - \text{intervention 2)}}$$

The ICER provides information about the amount of money to be spent for additional treatment in order to gain extra benefit.

9.2.4 Cost-utility analysis

The cost-utility analysis is a type of cost-effectiveness analysis which compares the cost of health care with its utility measured in QALYs. The QALY is a

9

single index of health benefit that includes quality and quantity of life and represents the outcome in a more comprehensive way than the single outcome, dependent cost-effectiveness analysis, that was discussed above.

You calculate the ICER by dividing the cost difference by the benefit difference, the latter measured in QALYs (see formula below). The QALYs could be determined, for example, by using the SF-36, SF-12 or Euroquol EQ5D.

$$ICER = \frac{\text{Difference in cost (intervention 1 – intervention 2)}}{\text{Difference in QALY (intervention 1 – intervention 2)}}$$

Let's go back to the example of breast cancer patients and calculate the ICER within a cost-utility analysis:

Group of patients with breast cancer

Benefit

If they continue to receiving standard treatment they will live on average for 1 year and their quality of life will be 0.4 (0 or below = worst possible health, 1 = best possible health)

If they receive a complex CAM intervention in addition to the standard treatment they will live for 1 year and 3 months (1.25 years), with a quality of life of 0.5.

Standard treatment: 1 year of extra life × 0.4 = 0.4 QALY

Standard treatment plus additional treatment: 1.25 years extra life × 0.5 = 0.625 QALYs

Therefore, the additional CAM intervention leads to 0.225 additional QALYs (0.625–0.4 QALY = 0.225 QALYs).

Costs

The cost of the standard treatment is 10,000 €. The cost of the standard treatment plus the additional CAM intervention is 13,000 €.

Incremental Cost Effectiveness Ratio (ICER)

The difference in treatment costs (3,000 €) is divided by the QALYs difference (0.225) to calculate the costs per QALY. So the additional CAM intervention would cost 13,333 € per QALY.

At the National Institute of Clinical Excellence (NICE) in the UK each intervention is considered on a case-by-case basis. Generally if a treatment costs more than £ 20,000–30,000 per additional QALY it is not considered cost-effective. www.nice.org.uk/newsroom/features/measuringeffectivenessandcost-effectivenesstheqaly.jsp (January 2010)

9.2.5 Cost-minimization analysis

The cost-minimization analysis is also a subcategory of the cost-effectiveness analysis. It compares the costs of achieving a given outcome by different procedures. This approach is used when the outcomes of the procedures being considered are known to be equal, and focuses on the identification of the cheapest cost option. Cost minimization should only be done when there is very high confidence that the outcomes are the same. This may be the case if previous studies have measured a non-inferiority or equivalence of treatments A and B. The following box gives an example of a cost-minimization analysis:

Example

In two groups of patients it was shown that qigong exercises were non-inferior to exercise therapy in improving chronic neck pain.

The cost of qigong intervention was 120 € whereas the cost of the exercise therapy was 90 €.

The exercise therapy resulted in lower costs.

9.3 Examples of economic analysis

Within the field of CAM most cost-effectiveness analyses have been published for acupuncture. They come mainly from Germany and the UK. The first from the United Kingdom (Wonderling et al. 2004) found acupuncture to be more cost-effective than conventional routine care.

All cost-effectiveness studies from Germany have shown that acupuncture is associated with better outcomes than usual care, but incurs additional costs. The German studies took a societal approach and calculated total and diagnosis specific costs. The total cost per QALY varied according to the diagnosis. It was between 3,000 €/QALY for dysmenorrhoea (Witt et al. 2008) and 18,000 €/QALY for osteoarthritis of the knee or the hip (Reinhold et al. 2008). The costs/QALY for low back pain (Witt et al. 2006), neck pain (Willich et al. 2006) and headache (Witt et al. 2008) were ranked somewhere in between. It would be interesting to see whether acupuncture might help to save costs in the long-term. The German cost-effectiveness studies lack such an analysis, whereas the study on low back pain from the United Kingdom (Ratcliffe et al. 2006) stretched over a period of two years. Here, the costs for the additional acupuncture treatment were not compensated by other savings after 2 years. Based on the available data we can currently assume that additional acupuncture treatment is associated with a higher benefit for the patients but also with higher costs for the purchasers.

As an example the cost evaluation of dysmenorrhea will be presented in more detail in the following box (Witt et al. 2008).

Cost evaluation of dysmenorrhea

Objective: To investigate the clinical effectiveness and cost-effectiveness of acupuncture in patients with dysmenorrhea.

Methods: In a randomized controlled trial with an additional non-randomized cohort, patients with dysmenorrhea were randomized to acupuncture (15 sessions over three months) or to a control group (no acupuncture). Patients who declined randomization received acupuncture treatment. All subjects were allowed to receive usual medical care.

The cost perspective was societal. Data analysis included

- 1) the overall costs during the 3 months after randomization (including costs not related to dysmenorrhea) and
- 2) only diagnosis-specific costs using ICD-10 codes to identify costs due to dysmenorrhea and related conditions.

Direct health-related costs for physician visits, hospital stays, medication, acupuncture treatment, and the number of days of sick leave were provided by the participating health insurance companies and valued using the human-capital approach. Cost per acupuncture session was € 35. Because the observation period was only 6 months in length, there was no need to discount any costs or effects. We compared costs between the 2 randomized groups and performed a cost-effectiveness analysis based on QALYs (cost-benefit analysis). The SF-36 data at baseline and after 3 months were transformed to the SF-6D using the algorithm developed by Brazier. Only patients with complete SF-36 data were included in the cost-effectiveness analysis. The analysis was based on the utility values at each time point using the common assumption of a linear change over time.

Results: For all 201 randomized patients (n = 201), we observed significant differences between the acupuncture and control group for the period between baseline to 3 months in overall costs (€ 666.66 [SD: 739.95] vs € 407.40 [SD: 1179.71], P < .001) and diagnosis-specific costs (€ 467.62 [SD: 401.20] vs € 29.95 [SD 76.05], P < .001). The mean difference between the two treatment groups during the 3 months intervention phase (overall: € 259.26, 95 % CI € 14.37, 532.89; diagnosis-specific: € 437.67, 95 % CI € 357.16, 518.18) was essentially due to the costs of acupuncture (€ 365.59 [SD: 98.56]) in the acupuncture group. Complete data on quality adjusted life years were available for 177 of the 201 randomized patients (88 %; 88 acupuncture, 89 control). As a result, only these 177 patients were included in the cost-effectiveness analysis. There were no significant differences between the two randomized groups at baseline (P = .085). Three months after randomization, QALY utility values were higher in the acupuncture group than in the control group (0.79 [SD: 0.11] vs 0.69 [SD: 0.13], P < .001). The cost difference between both groups was € 195.40 (SD: 152.33) for the overall costs and € 426.11 (SD: 43.39) for diagnosis-specific costs. The incremental cost effectiveness ratio was estimated to be € 3,011 per additional QALY gained (bootstrapped mean € 3,296, 95 % CI: € 1,705, 9025) in the overall cost perspective and € 6,567 (bootstrapped mean € 7,104, 95 % CI € 4,207, 12,679) in the diagnosis- specific cost perspective.

Conclusion: Additional acupuncture in patients with dysmenorrhoea was associated with improvements in quality of life as compared to treatment with usual care alone and was cost-effective within usual thresholds.

9.4 Critical appraisal

It is challenging that there is substantial variation in data and methods for health care cost evaluation across studies, and this applies even to studies with a seemingly similar intent. It is thus important to understand the context and the methods of each study.

In addition, mislabeling may result in considerable consequences, e.g. the labeling of partial evaluations as full economic evaluations has the potential to misinform the health care decision-making process. It may also result in the incorrect application of indexing terms to studies indexed for bibliographic databases (through no fault of the indexer!) – thus making it more challenging to identify studies containing true economic evaluations (Zarnke et al. 1997).

!

Take note that the results of cost-effectiveness analyses are valid mainly for the country where the study was performed. They are based on the relevant national health system, the local costs of the treatments, the assumptions on which the analysis is based (e.g. societal or third party payer perspective), and thus such studies may vary considerably between countries (Reinhold T et al.). These factors make the field of economic analysis more complicated than other areas of medical research.

When reading a publication of an economic evaluation you should check for the following aspects given in the 10 point checklist by Drummond et al. (2005).

Drummond's checklist for assessing economic evaluations

1. Was a well-defined question posed in answerable form?

1.1. Did the study examine both costs and effects of the service(s) or program(s)?

1.2. Did the study involve a comparison of alternatives?

1.3. Was a viewpoint for the analysis stated and was the study placed in any particular decision-making context?

2. Was a comprehensive description of the competing alternatives given (i.e. can you tell who did what to whom, where, and how often)?

2.1. Were there any important alternatives omitted?

2.2. Was (should) a do-nothing alternative (be) considered?

3. Was the effectiveness of the program or services established?

3.1. Was this done through a randomized, controlled clinical trial? If so, did the trial protocol reflect what would happen in regular practice?

3.2. Was effectiveness established through an overview of clinical studies?

3.3. Were observational data or assumptions used to establish effectiveness? If so, what are the potential biases in results?

4. Were all the important and relevant costs and consequences for each alternative identified?

4.1. Was the range wide enough for the research question at hand?

4.2. Did it cover all relevant viewpoints? (Possible viewpoints include the community or social viewpoint, and those of patients and third-party payers. Other viewpoints may also be relevant depending upon the particular analysis.)

4.3. Were the capital costs, as well as operating costs, included?

5. Were costs and consequences measured accurately in appropriate physical units (e.g. hours of nursing time, number of physician visits, lost work-days, gained life years)?

5.1. Were any of the identified items omitted from measurement? If so, does this mean that they carried no weight in the subsequent analysis?

5.2. Were there any special circumstances (e.g., joint use of resources) that made measurement difficult? Were these circumstances handled appropriately?

6. Were the cost and consequences valued credibly?

6.1. Were the sources of all values clearly identified? (Possible sources include market values, patient or client preferences and views, policy-makers' views and health professionals' judgments)

6.2. Were market values employed for changes involving resources gained or depleted?

6.3. Where market values were absent (e.g. volunteer labour), or market values did not reflect actual values (such as clinic space donated at a reduced rate), were adjustments made to approximate market values?

6.4. Was the valuation of consequences appropriate for the question posed (i.e. has the appropriate type or types of analysis – cost-effectiveness, cost-benefit, cost-utility – been selected)?

7. Were costs and consequences adjusted for differential timing?

7.1. Were costs and consequences that occur in the future 'discounted' to their present values?

7.2. Was there any justification given for the discount rate used?

8. Was an incremental analysis of costs and consequences of alternatives performed?

8.1. Were the additional (incremental) costs generated by one alternative over another compared to the additional effects, benefits, or utilities generated?

9. Was allowance made for uncertainty in the estimates of costs and consequences?

9.1. If data on costs and consequences were stochastic (randomly determined sequence of observations), were appropriate statistical analyses performed?

9.2. If a sensitivity analysis was employed, was justification provided for the range of values (or for key study parameters)?

9.3. Were the study results sensitive to changes in the values (within the assumed range for sensitivity analysis, or within the confidence interval around the ratio of costs to consequences)?

10. Did the presentation and discussion of study results include all issues of concern to users?

10.1. Were the conclusions of the analysis based on some overall index or ratio of costs to consequences (e.g. cost-effectiveness ratio)? If so, was the index interpreted intelligently or in a mechanistic fashion?

10.2. Were the results compared with those of others who have investigated the same question? If so, were allowances made for potential differences in study methodology?

10.3. Did the study discuss the generalizability of the results to other settings and patient/client groups?

10.4. Did the study allude to, or take account of, other important factors in the choice or decision under consideration (e.g. distribution of costs and consequences, or relevant ethical issues)?

10.5. Did the study discuss issues of implementation, such as the feasibility of adopting the 'preferred' program given existing financial or other constraints, and whether any freed resources could be redeployed to other worthwhile programs?

REFERENCES

Drummond MF, Sculpher MJ, Torrance GW. O'Brien BJ, Stoddard GL. Methods for the Economic Evaluation of Health Care Programmes. 3rd ed. 2005. Oxford: Oxford University Press.

Lipscomb et al. Health Care Costing: Data, Methods, Current Applications Medical Care. Volume 47, Number 7 Suppl 1, July 2009.

Mooney G, Russell EM, Weir RD. Choices for health care: a practical introduction to the economics of health care provision. London: Macmillian, 1986.

Ratcliffe J, Thomas KJ, MacPherson H, Brazier J. A randomised controlled trial of acupuncture care for persistent low back pain: cost effectiveness analysis. *BMJ* 2006;333(7569):626–628A.

Reinhold T, Brüggenjürgen B, Schlander M, Rosenfeld S, Hessel F, Willich SN. Economic Analysis Based on Multinational Studies – Methods for Adapting Findings to National Contexts. Journal of Public Health, accepted.

Reinhold T, Witt CM, Jena S, Brinkhaus B, Willich SN. Quality of life and cost-effectiveness of acupuncture treatment in patients with osteoarthritis pain. *Eur J Health Econ* 2008;9(3):209–19.

Sassi F. Calculating QALYs, comparing QALY and DALY calculations Health Policy and Planning 2006 21(5):402–408; doi:10.1093/heapol/czl018.

Ware JE, Sherbourne CD. The MOS 36-item short-form health survey (SF-36). I. Conceptual framework and item selection. Med Care 1992;30(6):473–83.220–3.

Williams A. Priority setting in public and private health care. A guide through the ideological jungle. Journal of Health Economics 1988;7:17,383.

Willich SN, Reinhold T, Selim D, Jena S, Brinkhaus B, Witt CM. Cost-effectiveness of acupuncture treatment in patients with chronic neck pain. *Pain* 2006;125(1–2):107–13.

Witt CM, Jena S, Selim D, Brinkhaus B, Reinhold T, Wruck K *et al*. Pragmatic randomized trial evaluating the clinical and economic effectiveness of acupuncture for chronic low back pain. *Am J Epidemiol* 2006;164(5):487–96.

Witt CM, Reinhold T, Brinkhaus B, Roll S, Jena S, Willich SN. Acupuncture in patients with dysmenorrhea: a randomized study on clinical effectiveness and cost-effectiveness in usual care. *Am J Obstet Gynecol* 2008;198(2):166–8.

Witt CM, Reinhold T, Jena S, Brinkhaus B, Willich SN. Cost-effectiveness of acupuncture treatment in patients with headache. *Cephalalgia* 2008;28(4):334–45)

Wonderling D, Vickers AJ, Grieve R, McCarney R. Cost effectiveness analysis of a randomised trial of acupuncture for chronic headache in primary care. *BMJ* 2004;328(7,442):747–9.

Zarnke KB, Levine MAH, O'Brien BJ. Cost-benefit analyses in the health-care literature: don't judge a study by its label. *Journal of Clinical Epidemiology* 1997;50:813–822.

FURTHER READING

Drummond MF, Sculpher MJ, Torrance GW. O'Brien BJ, Stoddard GL. Methods for the Economic Evaluation of Health Care Programmes. 3rd ed. 2005. Oxford: Oxford University Press.

CHAPTER

10 Single-case research

This chapter provides an introduction into methods investigating treatment effects in single patients.

10.1 Why case reports are not scientific

Throughout this book we are refering almost exclusively to studies in groups of patients. But it is the individual patient who is at the centre of health care. The description of individual cases is probably the most important didactic tool for teaching in medicine. It is highly impressive to hear a patient's personal story, to see his personal pattern of signs and symptoms, and what happened when he or she received treatment. Proponents of CAM treatments typically refer to reports of individual cases to show the benefits of their method. But why can such case reports contribute very little to proving scientifically that a treatment is effective?

Most case reports are retrospective accounts of an impressive case as perceived and documented by a provider. They serve to demonstrate a problem or the solution of a problem. They should be exemplary and bring the relevant clinical issues to the point. An interesting case will remain in our memory, and if we see a similar patient in practice we remember the crucial points to take care of. Sometimes observations in single cases can also generate new hypotheses or identify new treatment options.

But case reports are a problem from a scientific point of view since there is no explicit question with an open answer. Instead an evident treatment effect is demonstrated. Those who hear or read case reports are often already believers of the treatment in question or they have at least an open attitude towards the presented treatment. Imagine a convinced provider who is reporting a fabulous cure of a patient with advanced cancer. With only a slightly sceptical mind you will immediately come up with a number of questions: Did the patient truly suffer from advanced cancer? Was the patient truly cured? If so, did he/she receive other treatments which might have contributed to the cure? Could it have been a spontaneous remission? Only very rarely does the information provided in traditional single case reports sufficiently answer such questions.

!

Scientific single-case studies on treatment effects must ask (self-)critical questions. The two most fundamental questions are:
1) Is my observation reliable?
2) Which factors other than my treatment may explain the observed outcome?

10.2 Why single-case research is important

There is quite a lot of literature in CAM criticizing randomized controlled trials, and the relevance of single cases for clinical practice is often emphasized. But surprisingly, the number of systematic single-case studies performed in CAM is small. We believe that this is a pity because such research could contribute considerably to a critical evaluation of CAM therapies. Furthermore, although the workload associated with high-quality single-case studies must not be underestimated single case studies are probably the most feasible research tool for the busy practitioner.

Can the effectiveness of a CAM therapy be proven by single cases? Yes and no. In principle, it is possible to show a causal treatment effect in a single patient with a rigorous single-case study (➤ Ch. 10.3). However, showing that a treatment is generally effective in a given condition is not possible (unless there are consistent results from a large number of similar case studies).

Single-case studies are great instruments to improve the ability for (self-)critical observation. They can be used to generate hypotheses, to carefully observe and to analyze clinical processes. They can be used in quality assessments and serve as teaching material. It is unlikely that case studies will provide evidence that will convince sceptics, but open clinicians may listen carefully. If a large number of high quality single-case studies would become available combined analysis may provide further insights.

In summary, it would be unrealistic to expect that single-case studies could revolutionize CAM research – but they may well contribute important pieces in an evidence puzzle.

10.3 Assessing causality in single cases

There are two main methods to show or suggest causal relationships in single-cases studies: Randomized single-case experiments analyzed with statistical methods and figural correspondence.
Randomized single-case experiments will be discussed in ➤ chapter 10.4. Here we focus on figural correspondence.

This methodological concept has been elaborated mainly by Kiene (Kiene and von Schön-Angerer 1998, Kiene 2000; see also Teut 2009 for a brief summary) based on Dunckers (1935) 'Gestalt' approach. Gestalt is a characteristic configuration of patterns and elements which is unique to a phenomenon as a whole. Duncker argued that under certain circumstances the Gestalt of a cause can be perceived through the resulting effect. Kiene and von-Schön-Angerer cite as a simple example a car driving across a field leaving tracks that have the same surface structure as the tires. In this situation we do not need multiple randomized observations to be certain that it was the tire moving across the field that caused the tracks.

Kiene and von Schön-Angerer propose a set of criteria focussing on correspondence which allows to assess causality in the therapeutic process in single patients. **Time-figure correspondence** means that the observable effects of a therapeutic intervention correspond with a time pattern. For example, after the start and with continued treatment there is a steady improvement, when the treatment is disrupted there is clear symptom aggravation, and the pattern can be reproduced several times. If an ointment is applied to the skin of a patient suffering from a regionalized skin eruption in an S-shaped curve resulting in skin healing exactly in the S-shaped area treated, this is called **space-figure correspondence**. If the observed reaction after an intervention exactly corresponds with antomical structures (for example, in case of anesthetic nerve blocks or intraspinal anesthesia) this can be considered as **morphological correspondence**. If the size of the effect correponds with changes in the dose there is **dose-effect correspondence**. **Process-correspondence** means that changes in a complex therapeutic process follow a predicted temporal and structural pattern. The likelihood of a causal relationship is also increased if the **pre/post-time-relation** is large, that is if long-standing symptoms improve immediately after starting the treatment. Further indicators of a potential causal relationship include an effect size exceeding clearly what could be expected by chance, or what was observed during previous unsuccessful therapies. The more criteria are fulfilled in a single case the higher is the likelihood of a causal relationship.

We think that the concept of figural correspondence is important and fits very well to how clinicans think. However, we warn from unwarranted overoptimism. We are concerned that a careful analysis of most cases in routine care will show that very often effects and correspondence are not very clear and that the assessment of single causality criteria is difficult.

10.4 Experimental single-case studies

10.4.1 General aspects

In this book we define as experimental single case studies those in which the treatment strategy is modified for scientific purposes, for example, the number, duration and frequency of treatment sessions are predefined. If in an individual clinical situation the treatment is exclusively based on the clinician's (and hopefully the patient's) decision we consider the approach observational, even if a study includes elements which serve scientific purposes (for example, a systematic outcome measurement or diagnostic procedure which would not have been used in routine practice).

There is a considerable size of literature on experimental single-case studies in clinical psychology including valuable textbooks (e.g. Petermann & Müller 2001; Julius et al. 2000, Franklin et al. 1997). Experimental single-case studies typically share two characteristics: firstly, they consist of several predefined treatment and/or observation phases which are often desginated as phases A, B, C, etc. (➤ Fig. 10.1a). We propose to differentiate progressive and repetitive approaches. Secondly, the analysis is focusing on a quantitative or graphical comparison of the different phases often using specific statistical methods (single-case statistics). The sequence or timing of the treatment or observation periods may be non-randomized or randomized.

If you aim to perform an experimental single-case study in which you do not provide your treatmwent as you would normally do you should go for ethical approval.

10.4.2 Progressive approaches

Most basic experimental single-case studies follow an AB or an ABC design (➤ Fig. 10.1a), where A is a pre-assessment phase (or treatment 1), B the treatment phase (or treatment 2), and C a follow-up phase (or treatment 3). The following box summarizes an example. We call the approach progressive because single phases follow each other without being repeated. There can be more complex progressive approaches in which, for example, there is a second intervention phase (B') and a second follow-up phase (C'), to investigate whether effects are lasting. Progressive approaches can be applied in almost any chronic condition without interfering much with routine practice. The obvious limitation of such an approach is that due to the lack of alternating the different phases repeatedly it is not possible to assess whether effects are reproducible.

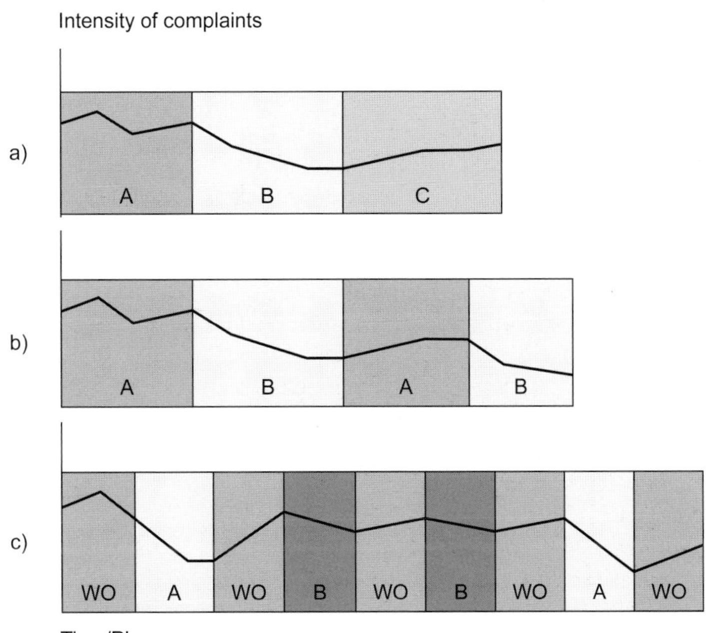

Fig. 10.1 Basic designs of experimental single-case studies: a) ABC design; b) ABAB design; c) Variable phases with wash-out (WO) periods in between

Example of a single-case study using an ABC design

Lee et al. (2005) observed a 35-year old man with advanced lung cancer (stage IV, metastases in stomach and bone) treated with radiotherapy and chemotherapy six months before, currently receiving only morphines for pain. At study entry his general condition was bad (Karnofsky Performance Scale 40, constantly high pain levels) requiring special care and assistance over the previous month. After six days of pre-treatment observation, the patient received eight sessions Korean external Qigong therapy on alternate days over 16 days, followed by a two-week post-treatment obervation phase. A variety of symptoms were assessed repeatedly using a visual analogue scale. The results were presented graphically (➤ Fig. 10.2).

Comment: The study shows convincingly that the patient improved. After initiation of Qigong treatment symptoms improved fast, consistently and distinctively. Improvements seem to persist in the short follow-up phase. A main weakness is the short pre-treatment observation period with only two measurements which leaves some uncertainty whether symptoms at study entry were particularly bad increasing the likelihood of regression to the mean or spontaneous improvement (although the authors report that the patient felt bad at least for the previous month).

It is possible to introduce a random element into such a study by randomizing, for example, how long the pre-treatment phase lasts and when the treatment starts (Schulte and Walach 2006). This to some

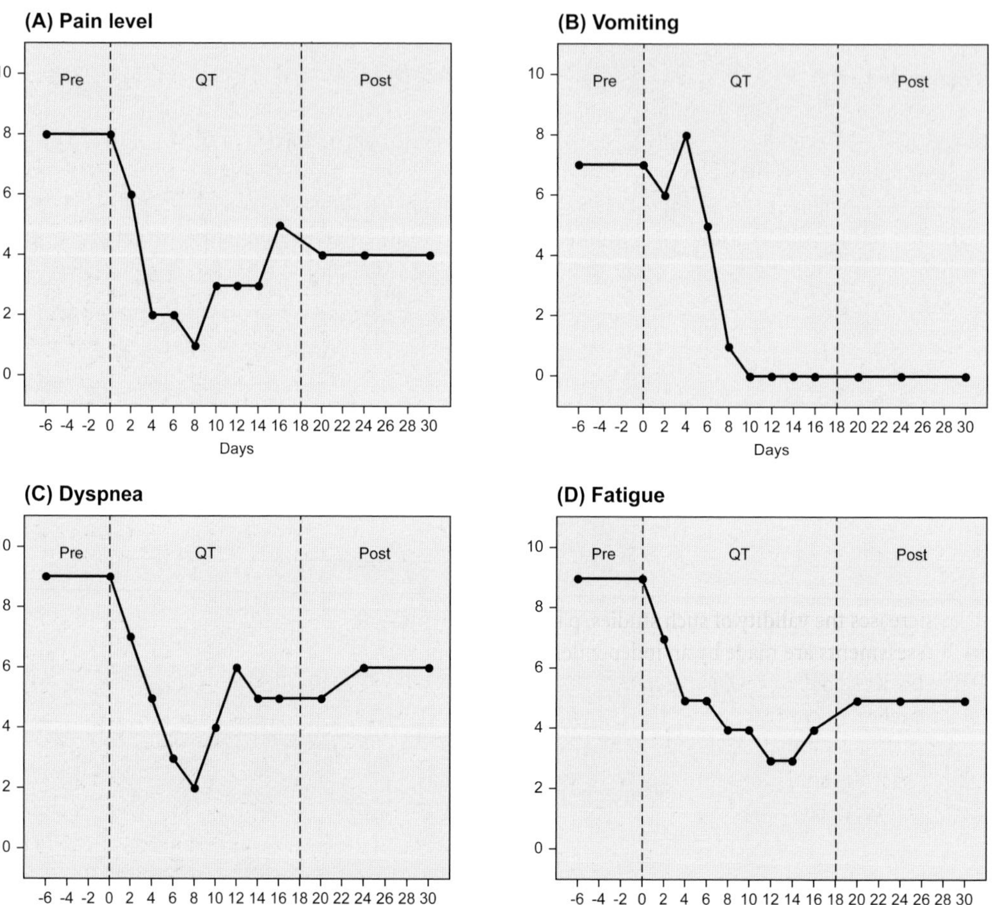

Fig. 10.2a Experimental single-case study using an ABC design by Lee et al. 2005. Display of ratings on visual analogue scales (y-axes) for (A) pain, (B) vomiting, (C) dyspnoe, (D) fatigue, (E) anorexia, (F) insomnia, (G) daily activities and (H) psychological calmness before treatment (pre), during external Qigong therapy (QT) and after treatment (post). Copyright Blackwell

10

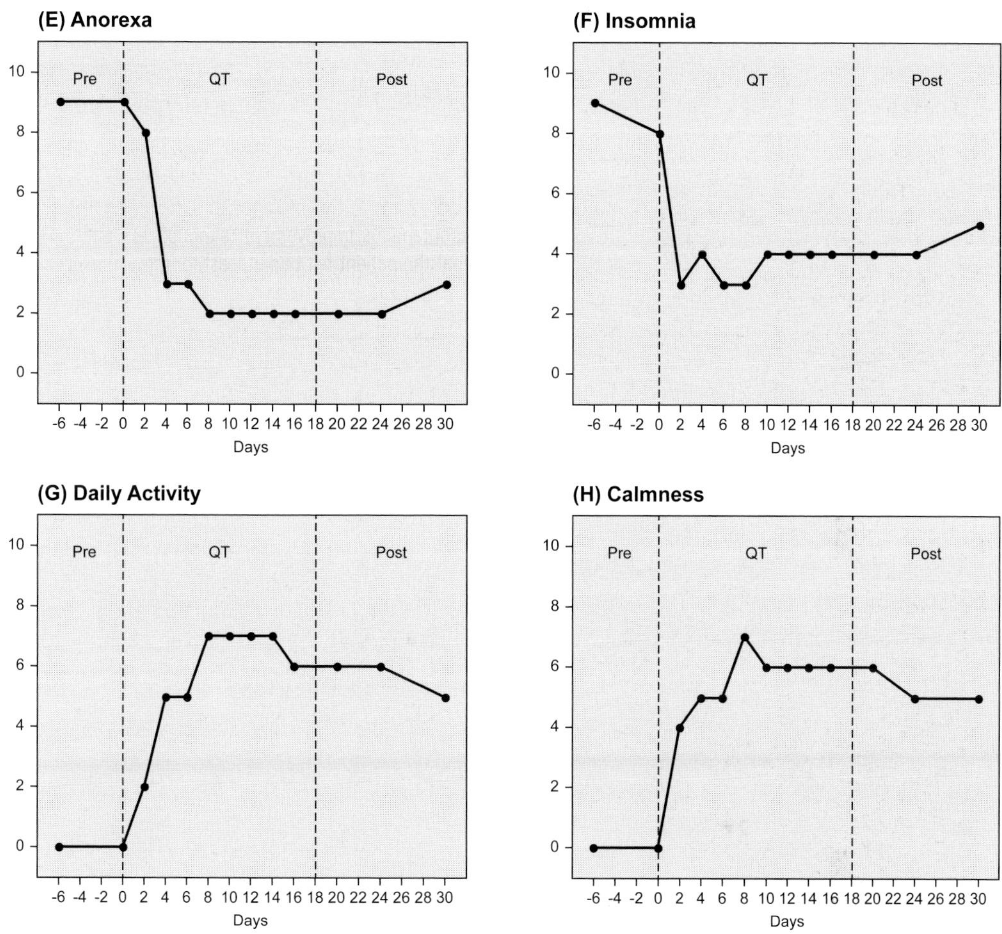

Fig. 10.2b Experimental single-case study using an ABC design by Lee et al. 2005. Display of ratings on visual analogue scales (y-axes) for (A) pain, (B) vomiting, (C) dyspnoe, (D) fatigue, (E) anorexia, (F) insomnia, (G) daily activities and (H) psychological calmness before treatment (pre), during external Qigong therapy (QT) and after treatment (post). Copyright Blackwell

extent increases the validity of such studies, particularly if assessments are made by an independent observer who does not know when the treatment starts, or if a placebo intervention is used during the baseline phase. If several such studies are combined to a multiple-baseline study (➢ Ch. 10.6.2) the conclusiveness increases considerably.

10.4.3 Repetitive approaches

If a patient suffers from a chronic condition and symptoms re-appear in the same intensity shortly after disrupting a treatment repetitive approaches are possible. If, for example, a patient with chronic pain receives the short acting analgesic A for three days he might have less pain during that time but after stopping the intake the pain comes back. He then could try analgesic B in the same way. If this is repeated once again in a study this is described as an ABAB design (➢ Fig. 10.1b). Depending on the number and sequence of treatments a variety of designs are possible (ABBA, ABBABAAB, etc.). If necessary wash-out phases have to be included if treatments have longer-lasting effects (➢ Fig. 10.1c). Several statistical methods are available to analyze repetitive single-case studies (Petermann & Müller 2001; Julius et al. 2000, Franklin et al. 1997).

The conclusiveness of such a repetitive study can be enhanced greatly if the multiple treatment phases are randomized. Then such a study is called a **n-of-1 trial**. If possible a n-of-1 trial is also blinded. In the following box one of the few examples of n-of-1 trials in CAM is summarized.

One of the main obstacles precluding the more frequent use of repetitive designs in general and n-of-1 trials in particular is that they can only be performed if the treatment does not have long-lasting effects and the condition is stable. In reality these two conditions are rarely met. Therefore, even though being methodologically preferable repetitive approaches can be used only rarely while the methodologically weaker progressive approaches are more feasible.

Example of a randomized n-of-1trial

Estrada & Young (1993) performed a double-blinded multiple cross-over placebo-controlled trial in a 61-year-old African-American male who had experienced side effects with several antihypertensive medications and was not willing to try others. The patient received three treatment pairs (each single phase three weeks) of a garlic-smelling placebo or a garlic preparation in randomized order. To provide a washout period, data from the first week after each cross-over were not included in the statistical analysis.

While the patient was taking garlic the mean systolic blood pressure was 146.9 mm compared to 148.9 under placebo ($p < 0.05$), the mean diastolic blood pressure was 87.2 vs. 89.6 ($p < 0.05$). The patient identified the capsule he was taking in 75% of the weeks. After reviewing the results of the study the patient insisted on receiving only garlic for the management of his hypertension in spite of the small effect.

Comment: While unblinding might have introduced some bias the study suggests that there was a small blood pressure lowering effect of the garlic treatment.

10

10.5 Observational single case studies

10.5.1 Retrospective case studies

Observational single case studies are scientificially less conclusive than experimental single case studies, however, as they do not interfer or interfer only very little with what you normally do in practice they are easier to perform. Furthermore, while you should always obtain written informed consent from the patient in many countries you will not need approval from an ethical review board.

If you have a very good documentation it will be possible in some situations to do a rigorous case analysis retrospectively. For example, some cancer centers have detailed routine documentation and follow patients over long periods of time. If you see a case which is really unusual (a "best case") it might be worthwhile to analyse it in detail. Retrospective case studies are valuable only if your documentation allows to credibly answer the questions raised in ➤ Ch. 10.1: Did the patient truly suffer from advanced cancer? Did the patient truly improve? If so, did he receive other treatments? Could it have been a spontaneous remission? In oncology a checklist has been published giving recommendations for details to be included in high quality (retrospective) case studies (Kienle et al. 2004).

10.5.2 Prospective case studies

From a methodological point of view it is much better to follow a case prospectively. Before actually starting the treatment you decide with the patient that you will follow him/her accurately and systematically. It makes sense to clearly formulate objectives you want to reach with the treatment, to verify the clincial diagnosis according to the highest standard, and to carefully document the course of disease in the last hours, days or months – with time frames decided appropriate to the condition. You should use validated instruments for measuring symptoms, signs, quality of life, etc. before starting the treatment and predefine when you will use them again. In addition, you should carefully document all important observations before, during and after treatment as needed. Take care that you make sure that several perspectives (patient, provider, possibly also relatives) are reflected in your documentation. Detail and consistency increase the conclusiveness more than anything else. Yor are free to treat as you would treat outside of the study, but document carefully. An example of a prospective case study is provided in the following box.

The main drawback of prospective case studies is that you have to decide in advance whether you will study a patient. It might be that this patient turns out to be non-compliant or that the course of disease in this patient is worse than in the patients you treat usually. The likelihood of having selected a patient which is not a best case is high.

Example of a prospective observational single-case study

Teut and Warning (2008) prospectively observed an 87-year-old woman with severe joint pain due to osteoarthritis of the knee who presented with side effects from a potent pain killer (fentanyl). Together with the patient they chose pain intensity (using a numerical rating scale), walking distance and activites of daily living (measured with the Barthel index) as outcome measures. The patient was treated (in an in-patient setting) with leeches, herbal medicine, physiotherapy and three single doses of metamizol. Under therapy the patient experienced a clear reduction in pain (from 8 to 3 points on the numerical rating scale). She regained walking ability (increase in walking distance from 0 to 70 m) and showed improvements in the Barthel Index (from 45 to 65). Using criteria of figural correspondence several criteria suggested a causal treatment effect: there was a fast and marked improvement within a few days after complaints had been stable for about three months. The timing of improvement was predicted based on available evidence.
Comment: this is a carefully documented case-study which suggests a causal relationship between improvement and the treatment applied. However, it also shows how difficult it is in routine care to prove causaility beyond reasonable doubt.

10.5.3 Semi-prospective case studies

Semiprospective case studies could be a compromise balancing the advantages of retrospective case studies (focus on particularly interesting cases) and prospective case studies (systematic documentation). If early in the treatment process you become aware that a specific case may be of particular interest you carfully document what has happend so far and then start prospective documentation.

There are some cases in the literature where semi-prospective methods seem to have been used as the documentation is quite systematic. However, publications of such single-case studies rarely describe their methods in detail, so it is difficult to decide whether the approach was retrospective (based on a systematic high quality routine documentation) or semi-prospective (e.g. Wode et al. 2009).

10.6 Cross-roads between research on single cases and groups of patients

10.6.1 Best case series

A best case series is a documentation of a number of cases which have gone particularly well. If such a best case series is really indicating surprisingly positive outcomes in a number of individuals it can stimulate further and more systematic research. For example, the Office of Cancer Complementary and Alternative Medicine (OCCAM) of the US National Cancer Institute has launched a best case series program in oncology (www.cancer.gov/cam/bestcase_intro.html). Providers of CAM therapies are invited to submit their best cases. To be considered as conclusive, reports must meet stringent criteria. In case of the OCCAM program these are:

- 1) well-documented, definitive diagnosis of cancer;
- 2) an adequate documentation of disease response;
- 3) absence of confounders (no concurrent treatments with known therapeutic potential);
- 4) an adequately documented treatment history.

An example from such a best case series is summarized in box 4. Obviously, best case series can be performed for other conditions using adapted criteria.

10

Example of a best case series

Banerji et al. (2008) have published a report on a best case series evaluated in the program of the Office of Cancer Complementary and Alternative Medicine (OCCAM) of the US National Cancer Institute. Lung and oesophageal carcinoma patients were treated with homoeopathic remedies in an Indian centre according to a specific

(Banerji) protocol until there was complete regression of the tumors. Case records including pathology and radiology reports for 14 patients were submitted for review by the US NCI BCS Program. Four of these cases had an independent confirmation of the diagnosis and radiographic response and were accepted as sufficient information for the NCI to initiate further investigation. The results of the review were deemed to be sufficient to warrant an NCI-initiated prospective research follow-up in the form of an observational study.

10.6.2 Multiple baseline studies

Mutiple baseline studies with slightly variable approaches are quite frequently used in behavioral research (Barlow and Hersen 1984). For CAM research one variant seems of particular interest (> Fig. 10.3). Several patients are observed over a longer period with repeated measurement of the outcome of interest. In the first phase (baseline) they do not receive the treatment investigated. The duration of the baseline phase and the timing of the switch to the treatment phase are variable. If possible the timing of the switch is randomized and remains unknown to patient and treatment provider until the treatment is to be started. If in such a study a placebo can be used or if outcome measurements can be performed by a blinded independent observer, the validity of a multiple baseline study can be enhanced greatly. If a consistent response pattern with marked improvements after initiating treatment emerges, such designs can provide quite impressive preliminary evidence. Therefore, they are sometimes used as pilot studies for larger observational or experimental studies (see Keays et al. 2008 for an example on Pilates exercises and shoulder problems in women with breast cancer).

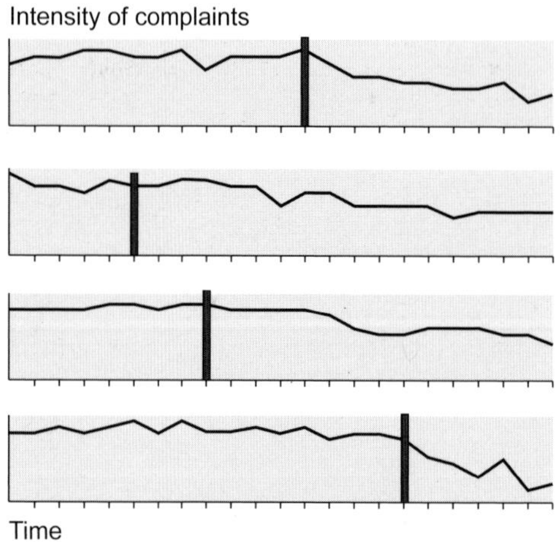

Fig. 10.3 Multiple baseline design: several patients are observed over a longer period of time with repeated measurements. The timing of the switch from baseline to treatment (fat lines) can be randomized

10.6.3 Single-case studies embedded in studies of groups of patients

It is possible to integrate single-case studies into observational or experimental studies in larger groups of patients. For example, Hamre et al. (2004) performed a prospective observational study of anthroposophic art therapy in 161 patients. Within the study intensity of complaints, quality of life, depressive symptoms, use of other treatments, satisfaction with treatment and a variety of other outcome measures were documented repeatedly up to 24 months after inclusion. Sixteen patients were selected for additional single case analysis for which additional interviews were performed. Using figural correspondence the authors tried to assess the likelihood of causality for the observed treatment effects. Walach et al. (2000) conducted a 1-year observational study of 18 patients with chronic headaches who had previously participated in a placebo-controlled randomized trial of classical homeopathy. Patients filled in diaries which were analyzed using single-case statistical methods.

Single-case studies embedded in studies of groups of patients can serve to collect additional qualitative information for a better understanding of processes, for a more detailed and individualized evaluation and possibly for strengthening the conclusiveness.

10.6.4 Meta-analysis of single-case studies

Published multiple single-case studies on the same condition using similar methodology can be summarized in a systematic review or a meta-analysis. To the best of our knowledge this has not yet been done in CAM due to the lack of a sufficient number of similar single case studies. However, what has been done already are series of randomized n-of-1 trials designed prospectively and in a manner to allow for their combined analysis (e.g. Coxeter et al. 2003).

REFERENCES

Banerjy P, Campbell DR, Banerji P. Cancer patients treated with the Banerji protocols using homoeopathic medicine: a best case series program of the National Cancer Institute USA. Oncology Rep 2008;20:69–74.

Barlow DH, Hersen M. Multiple baseline designs. In: Goldstein AP, Krasner L, eds. Single case experimental designs: strategies for studying behaviour change. New York: Pergamon Press, 1984:210–51.

Cowell IM, Philips DR. Effectiveness of manipulative physiotherapy for the treatment of a neurogenic cervicobrachial pain syndroms: a single cases study-experimental design. Man Ther 2002;7:31–38.

Coxeter PD, Schluter PJ, Eastwood HL, Nikles CJ, Glasziou P. Valerian does not appear to reduce symptoms for patients with chronic insomnia in general practice using a series of randomised n-of-1 trials. Complement Ther Med 2003;11:215–222.

Duncker K. Zur Psychologie des produktiven Denkens. Berlin: Springer, 1935.

Estrada CA, Young MJ. Patient preferences for novel therapy: an n-of-1 trial of garlic in the treatment of hypertension. J Gen Intern Med 1993;6:619–621.

Franklin RD, Allison DB, Gorman BS (eds). Design and analysis of single-case research. Mahwah: Lawrence Erlbaum Associates, 1997.

Hamre HJ, Glockmann A, Kiene H. Wirksamkeitsbeurteilung der Anthroposophischen Kunsttherapie: Einzelfallstudie eingebettet in eine prospektive Kohortenstudie. Merkurstab 2004;57:194–203.

Julius H, Schlosser RW, Goetze H. Kontrollierte Einzelfallstudien. Göttingen: Hogrefe, 2000.

Keays KS, Harris SR, Lucyshyn JM, MacIntyre DL. Effects of Pilates exercises on shoulder range of motion, pain, mood, and upper-extremity function in women living with breast cancer: a pilot study. Phys Ther 2008;88:494–510.

Kiene H, von Schön-Angerer T. Single-case causality assessment as a basis for clinical judgement. Alt Ther Health Med 1998;4:41–47.

Kiene H. Komplementäre Methodenlehre der klinischen Forschung. Cognition-based medicine. Berlin: Springer, 2000.

Kienle GS, Hamre HJ, Öportalupi E, Kiene H. Improving the quality of therapeutic reports of single cases and case series in oncology – criteria and checklist. Alt Ther Health Mded 2004;10:68–72.

Lee MS, Yang SH, Lee KK, Moon SR. Effects of Qi therapy (external Qigong) on symptoms of advanced cancer: a single case study. Eur J Cancer 2005;14:457–462.

Petermann F, Müller JM. Clinical psychology and single-case evidence – a practical approach to treatment, planning and evaluation. Chichester: Wiley, 2001.

Schulte D, Walach H. F.M. Alexander technique in the treatment of stuttering – a randomized single-case intervention study with ambulatory monitoring. Psychother Psychosom 2006;75: 190–191.

Teut M, Warning A. Blutegel, Phytotherapie und Physiotherapie bei Gonarthrose – eine geriatrische Fallstudie. Forsch Komplementärmed 2008;15:269–272.

Teut M. Scientific case studies in homeopathy. In: Witt C, Albrecht H (eds). New directions in homeopathy research. Essen: KVC Verlag, 2009, pp 67–79.

Walach H, Lowes T, Mussbach D, Schamell U, Springer W, Stritzl G, Haag U. The long-term effects of homeopathic treatment of chronic headaches: one year follow-up and single case time series analysis. Br Homeop J 2001;90:63–72.

Wode K, Schneider T, Lundberg I, Kienle GS. Mistletoe treatment in cancer-related fatigue: a case report. Cases Journal 2009, 2:77.

CHAPTER

11 A brief look at other study designs

This chapter provides short introductions to some other important research designs not covered in detail in this book.

11.1 Cross-sectional studies/ surveys

The study designs discussed so far are all longitudinal, that is, study participants are observed over an extended period of time. Studies which take "a picture" at one moment in time are called cross-sectional studies. The most typical type of cross-sectional study is a survey. Surveys can be used for a variety of purposes such as evaluating the use of CAM (Example 1), gathering information on training of providers (Example 2) or collecting data on adverse effects of CAM (Example 3).

Surveys – Example 1

Eisenberg DM, Kessler RC, Foster C, Norlock FE, Calkins DR, Delbanco TL. Unconventional medicine in the United States. Prevalence, costs, and patterns of use. N Engl J Med. 1993;328:246–52.

Background: Many people use unconventional therapies for health problems, but the extent of this use and the costs are not known. The authors conducted a national survey to determine the prevalence, costs, and patterns of use of unconventional therapies, such as acupuncture and chiropractic.

Methods: The study was limited to 16 commonly used interventions neither taught widely in U.S. medical schools nor generally available in U.S. hospitals. Telephone interviews with 1,539 adults (response rate, 67 percent) were completed in a national sample of adults 18 years of age or older in 1990. Respondents were asked to report any serious or bothersome medical conditions and details of their use of conventional medical services; they were then inquired about their use of unconventional therapy.

Results: 34 % of respondents reported using at least one unconventional therapy in the past year, and a third of these saw providers for unconventional therapy. The latter group had made an average of 19 visits to such providers during the preceding year, with an average charge per visit of \$ 27.60. The frequency of use of unconventional therapy varied somewhat among sociodemographic groups, with the highest use reported by nonblack persons from 25 to 49 years of age who had relatively more education and higher incomes. The majority used unconventional therapy for chronic, as opposed to life-threatening, medical conditions. Among those who used unconventional therapy for serious medical conditions, the vast majority (83 percent) also sought treatment for the same condition from a medical doctor; however, 72 percent of the respondents who used unconventional therapy did not inform their medical doctor that they had done so.

Conclusions: The frequency of use of unconventional therapy in the United States is far higher than previously reported. Medical doctors should ask about their patients' use of unconventional therapy whenever they obtain a medical history.

Surveys – Example 2

Sherman KJ, Cherkin DC, Kahn J, Erro J, Hrbek A, Deyo RA, Eisenberg DM. A survey of training and practice patterns of massage therapists in two US states. BMC Complement Altern Med. 2005;5:13.

Background: Despite the growing popularity of therapeutic massage in the US, little is known about the training or practice characteristics of massage therapists. This survey aimed to describe these characteristics.

Methods: As part of a study of random samples of complementary and alternative medicine (CAM) practitioners, 226 massage therapists licensed in Connecticut and Washington state were interviewed by telephone in 1998 and 1999 (85 % of those contacted) and then asked a sample of them to record information on 20 consecutive visits to their practices (total of 2005 consecutive visits).

Results: Most massage therapists were women (85 %), white (95 %), and had completed some continuing education training (79 % in Connecticut and 52 % in

Washington). They treated a limited number of conditions, most commonly musculoskeletal (59 % and 63 %) (especially back, neck, and shoulder problems), wellness care (20 % and 19 %), and psychological complaints (9 % and 6 %) (especially anxiety and depression). Practitioners commonly used one or more assessment techniques (67 % and 74 %) and gave a massage emphasizing Swedish (81 % and 77 %), deep tissue (63 % and 65 %), and trigger/pressure point techniques (52 % and 46 %). Self-care recommendations, including increasing water intake, body awareness, and specific forms of movement, were made as part of more than 80 % of visits. Although most patients self-referred to massage, more than one-quarter were receiving concomitant care for the same problem from a physician. Massage therapists rarely communicated with these physicians.
Conclusion: This study provides new information about licensed massage therapists that should be useful to physicians and other healthcare providers interested in learning about massage therapy in order to advise their patients about this popular CAM therapy.

There are probably only few CAM researchers who have never been involved in a cross-sectional study. As can be seen from these examples, there are plenty of approaches for surveys.

!

Although surveys seem to be relatively easy to perform, they should be planned and prepared carefully!

As for every study you should define your main objectives. These will form the basis for the questions you will ask in your survey. You can find information on the development of questions in ➢ chapter 4.8. After developing your questions you should conduct a pilot test to check if they are understandable and revise them if necessary. The selection of the population sample to test your questions depends on your objective. It is important that the selected sample is representative of the group you aim to do your survey on. A variety of methods can be used to perform the survey in practical terms, for example, questionnaires could be distributed by providers or they could be sent by mail to patients, telephone interviews could be performed, or the survey could be web based. The feasibility of your study will be determined by the type of population sample, the method of and manpower for questionnaire distribution, financial aspects, data management and data analysis and the accessibility of the sample.

Surveys – Example 3

Vohra S, Brulotte J, Le C, Charrois T, Laeeque H. Adverse events associated with paediatric use of complementary and alternative medicine: Results of a Canadian Paediatric Surveillance Program survey. Paediatr Child Health. 2009;14:385–7.

Background: Despite many studies confirming that the use of complementary and alternative medicine (CAM) by children is common, few have assessed related adverse events. We conducted a national survey to identify the frequency and severity of adverse events associated with paediatric CAM use.
Methods: Survey questions were developed based on a review of relevant literature and consultation with content experts. In January 2006, the Canadian Paediatric Surveillance Program distributed the survey to all paediatricians and paediatric subspecialists in active practice in Canada.
Results: Of the 2,489 paediatricians who received the survey, 583 (23 %) responded. Respondents reported that they asked patients about CAM use 38 % of the time and that patients disclosed this information before being questioned only 22 % of the time. Forty-two paediatricians (7 %) reported seeing adverse events, most commonly involving natural health products, in the previous year. One hundred five paediatricians (18 %) reported witnessing cases of delayed diagnosis or treatment (n = 488) that they attributed to the use of CAM.
Conclusion: While serious adverse events associated with paediatric CAM appear to be rare, delays in diagnosis or treatment seem more common. Given the lack of paediatrician-patient discussion regarding CAM use, our findings may under-represent adverse events. A lack of reported adverse events should not be interpreted as a confirmation of safety. Active surveillance is required to accurately assess the incidence, nature and severity of paediatric CAM-related adverse events. Patient safety demands that paediatricians routinely inquire about the use of CAM.

The main problem in surveys is participation. However in order to gain representative results it is important to achieve a high response rate. The response rate of 67 % in example 1 is a very good response rate for a nationwide survey, whereas the response rate of 23 % in example 3 is very low. A response rate of 23 % means that you have no information from more than three quarters of your population, thus the results are not representative. To ensure a high response rate think carefully about the selection of your sample, send reminders to those who did not answer and consider incentives.

11.2 Diagnostic studies

Diagnosis plays a fundamental role in any medical system. Without some kind of diagnostic classification it is impossible to decide on a treatment (unless you use one treatment for everything). In relation to the importance of diagnosis, diagnostic issues are clearly under-researched in all medicine, but particularly in CAM. There are several reasons for this, one being that diagnostic research is conceptually not easy. The most important types of diagnostic study are reliability studies and validity studies.

Reliability studies investigate whether several investigators independently reach the same conclusion when applying a diagnostic test (inter-rater reliability; ➤ Fig. 11.1), or whether the same investigator comes to the same conclusion at different times (intra-rater reliability).

A diagnostic test can be everything from a chiropractic assessment of the mobility of a defined vertebra to a homeopathic case taking. The main outcomes of reliability studies are measures of agreement beyond that expected by chance. Examples are the so-called kappa index or the intra class correlation coefficient. The majority of the limited number of diagnostic studies in CAM focuses on reliability – and to our knowledge findings have often been disappointing. For example, one study investigated interexaminer reliability of lumbar segmental mobility and pain provocation using 2 experienced clinicians performing 3 palpation procedures over the lumbar facet joints and sacroiliac joints (Example 4).

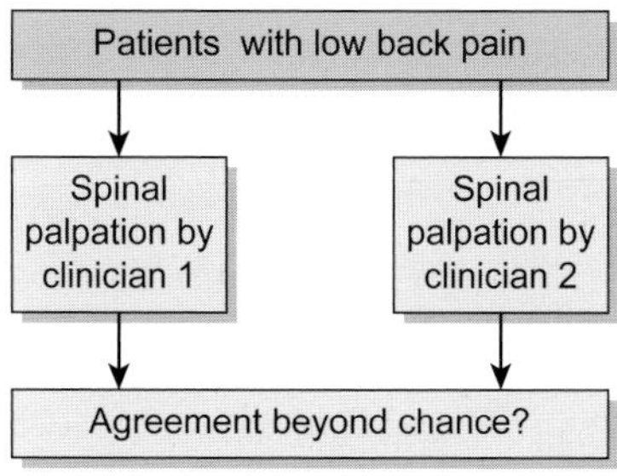

Fig. 11.1 Principle of a study of inter-rater-reliability – Example of a study on spinal palpation in patients with low back pain. All patients are assessed independently by two clinicians. Agreement between the two raters is then assessed involving statistical methods

Reliability study – Example 4

Schneider M, Erhard R, Brach J, Tellin W, Imbarlina F, Delitto A. Spinal palpation for lumbar segmental mobility and pain provocation: an interexaminer reliability study. J Manipulative Physiol Ther. 2008;31:465–73.

Objective: This study investigated the degree of interexaminer reliability using 2 experienced clinicians performing 3 palpation procedures over the lumbar facet joints and sacroiliac joints.

Methods: Study participants were 39 patients with low back pain. Two doctors of chiropractic independently examined each of these patients in the prone position with 3 different procedures: (1) springing palpation for pain provocation, (2) springing palpation for segmental mobility testing, and (3) the prone instability test. The doctors were blinded to each other's findings and the patient's clinical status, and performed the examinations on the same day. Standard and adjusted kappa values were calculated for each test.

Results: The kappa values for palpation of segmental motion restriction were poor (range, -.20 to .17) and in many cases less than chance observation (negative kappa values). The prone instability test showed reasonable reliability (kappa = .54), and palpation for segmental pain provocation also showed fair to good reliability (kappa range, .21 to .73).

Conclusions: Palpation methods that are used to provoke pain responses are more reliable than palpation methods in which the clinician purports to find segmental motion restriction. The prone instability test shows good reliability.

In principle, validity studies have more direct clinical importance but sufficient reliability should be established before embarking on a validity study.

Studies of diagnostic validity (or diagnostic accuracy) investigate whether a diagnostic procedure is helpful to rule in or rule out a diagnosis.

For example, in conventional medicine such studies investigate whether a simple new test such as the measurement of brain natriuretic peptide is useful to screen for heart failure in the elderly (➤ Fig. 11.2). In such a validity study the concen-

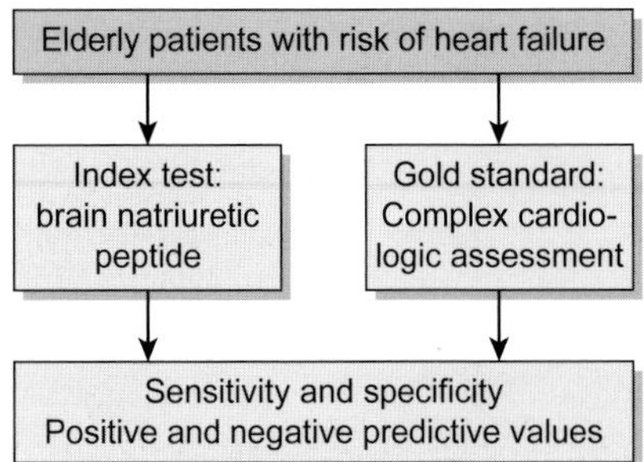

Fig. 11.2 Principle of a classical diagnostic validity study – Comparison of an index test (brain natriuretic peptide) with the gold standard (complex cardiologic assessment) to establish or rule out heart failure

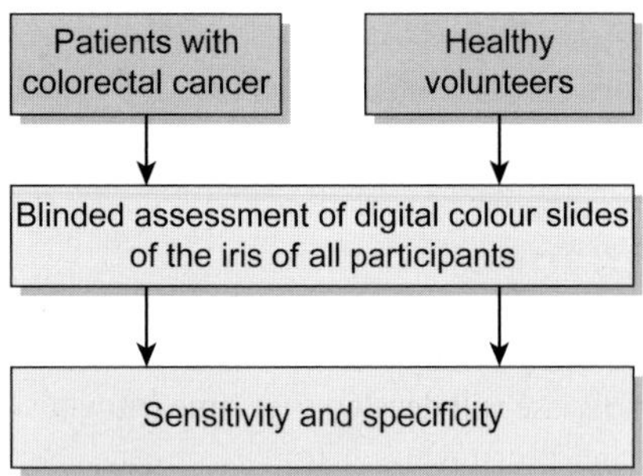

Fig. 11.3 Principle of a validity study (study on iridology) in which the diagnostic test is not used in a natural setting (patients in which the diagnosis is still to be made) but in a group of patients known to suffer from the disease and in a group of healthy controls

tration of brain natriuretic peptide would be measured in all patients included in the study (if possible this would be a representative sample of those who would undergo the test in routine practice). The diagnostic test of interest – in our example the measurement of brain natruretic peptide – is called the "index test". The diagnostic finding of this test would be compared with the "gold standard", the best available method of establishing whether heart failure is present or not. In case of heart failure this is a combination of symptoms and methods used by experienced cardiologists including typical clinical signs, and objective evidence of dysfunction as assessed by echocardiography or electrocardiography. The diagnostic tests have to be performed strictly independently in all patients. The classical finding of such studies are sensitivity (proportion of those classified ill with the new test among all individuals having the condition), specificity (proportion of those classified not ill among those not having the condition), positive and negative predictive value (if the test is positive or negative how likely the patient has the disease or does not have the disease, respectively).

Few validity studies have been performed on CAM methods. For example, there are a few studies on the diagnostic examination iridology. These studies did not find evidence that iridology is helpful in detecting cancer or inflammation of the gall bladder. The studies on iridology and other diagnostic validity studies in CAM usually use a design which is slightly different from the classical approach described above. For example, in one iridology study colour slides of the iris of a group of patients proven to suffer from colorectal cancer were compared with the slides taken from healthy volunteers (➤ Fig. 11.3 and example 5).

Diagnostic validity study – Example 5

Herber S, Rehbein M, Tepas T, Pohl C, Esser P. Looking for colorectal cancer in the patients iris? Ophthalmologe. 2008;105:570–4.

Background: Some authors claim that iridology is able to detect diseases by looking for abnormalities of pigmentation and structure in the iris. Our study investigated the applicability of iridology as an alternative screening method for colorectal cancer.

Methods: Digital color slides were obtained from both eyes of 29 patients with histologically diagnosed colorectal cancer and from 29 age- and gender-matched healthy control subjects. The slides were presented in random order to acknowledged iridologists without knowledge of the number of patients in the two categories.

Results: The iridologists correctly detected 51.7 % and 53.4 %, respectively, of the patients' slides; therefore, the likelihood was statistically no better than chance. Sensitivity was, respectively, 58.6 % and 55.2 %, and specificity was 44.8 % and 51.7 %.

Conclusions: In this study iridology had no validity as a diagnostic tool for detecting colorectal cancer.

11.3 Etiological and prognostic studies

Another important part of any medical system is concerning theories about the causes or risk factors for diseases (etiology). These are also relevant for predicting whether a disease will occur in the future or how a disease will develop over time (prognosis). Etiology and prognosis are classical research issues of epidemiology. There are plenty of etiological postulates in CAM which could be investigated. For example, traditional Chinese medicine has a complex theoretical system about pathogenetic factors. Or some CAM practitioners hold the belief that immunizations can increase the risk of developing allergic or other chronic diseases.

A classical etiological study is the case-control study (➤ Fig. 11.4 and example 6).

Case-control studies try to estimate the relative risk associated with a risk factor by investigating how many of the cases (individuals with the disease of interest) and how many of the controls (individuals without the disease) have been exposed to the risk factor.

This design is often difficult to understand for non-epidemiologists. A case-control study typically starts with the collection of cases. These are individuals who suffer from a specific disease, for example, children with diagnosed leukemia. Then the controls are selected. These should be children from the same population with similar age, sex, socio-economic status etc. – but who do not have leukaemia. After cases and controls have been selected the investigators then try to find out to what extent the individuals have been exposed to the risk factor of interest. The result of a case control study is typically expressed as an odds ratio ((number of cases who had been exposed/number of cases who had not been exposed)/(number of controls who had been exposed/number of cases who have not been exposed)). Remember that from this kind of retrospective study it is not possible to estimate the absolute risk that a person exposed to the risk factor develops the disease. You started with cases and controls: all cases have the disease and all controls do not have the disease. You can only find out whether or not exposure is more frequent in cases than in controls. Case-control studies are retrospective. They can be performed with limited resources, they are fast, and are also feasible if a condition is rare. A clear disadvantage is that exposure must be assessed retrospectively which provides plenty of room for inaccuracies and bias. Case-control studies could be applied well to etiological questions in CAM research.

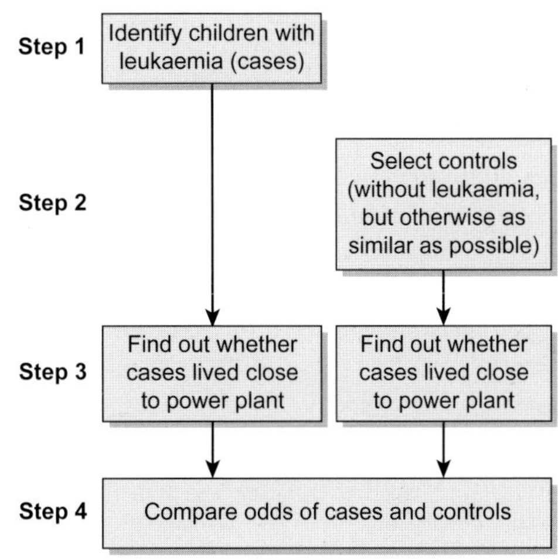

Fig. 11.4 Principle of a case-control study – Comparison of the odds of living close to a power plant among children with leukaemia (cases) and children without leukaemia

Case control study – Example 6

Malagoli C, Fabbi S, Teggi S, Calzari M, Poli M, Ballotti E, Notari B, Bruni M, Palazzi G, Paolucci P, Vinceti M. Risk of hematological malignancies associated with magnetic fields exposure from power lines: a case-control study in two municipalities of northern Italy. Environ Health. 2010;9:16.

Background: Some epidemiologic studies have suggested an association between electromagnetic field exposure induced by high voltage power lines and childhood leukemia, but null results have also been found and the possibility of bias due to unmeasured confounders has been suggested.

Methods: A case-control study was performed to study this relation in two municipalities of northern Italy, identifying the corridors along high voltage power lines with calculated magnetic field intensity in the 0.1-<0.2, 0.2-<0.4, and > or = 0.4 microTesla ranges. 64 cases of newly-diagnosed hematological malignancies in children aged <14 were identified within these municipalities

11

from 1986 to 2007. Four matched controls were sampled for each case, collecting information on historical residence and parental socioeconomic status of these subjects.
Results: The odds ratio of leukemia associated with antecedent residence in the area with exposure > or = 0.1 microTesla was 3.2 (6.7 adjusting for socioeconomic status), but this estimate was statistically very unstable, its 95 % confidence interval being 0.4–23.4, and no indication of a dose-response relation emerged. Relative risk for acute lymphoblastic leukemia was 5.3 (95 % confidence interval 0.7–43.5), while there was no increased risk for the other hematological malignancies.
Conclusions: Though the number of exposed children in this study was too low to allow firm conclusions, results were more suggestive of an excess risk of leukemia among exposed children than of a null relation.

The counterpart of case-control studies are cohort studies (➤ Fig. 11.5 and example 7). These are mostly prospective studies.

In a **cohort study** a large group of individuals is followed over a long period and their exposure to defined risk factors or their behaviour is documented to find out whether these factors have an influence on the risk of developing a specific disease or resulting in a defined outcome.

You start with a group of individuals who do not have the disease of interest, then you observe, usually over several years, whether your participants are exposed to a certain risk factor (for example, noise) or show a specific behaviour (for example, the extent to which women consume sweetened beverages), and whether they develop a disease or a health problem, e.g. experience a heart attack. Such studies allow both the estimation of absolute risks in case of a given behaviour, and a comparison of how outcomes differ between groups with different exposure or behavioural patterns. The main problems of cohort studies are that they have to be huge, take years to complete, and in consequence are very expensive. They are, in general, more reliable than case-control studies, however they suffer from the typical problems of any non-randomized comparison. Epidemiologists typically speak of confounding when other factors than the risk factor of interest are also associated with the outcome of interest.

Large cohort studies can also often provide prognostic information. For example, using data from large cohort studies, researchers have developed formulae which allow a prediction of the risk of having a heart attack within the next ten years based on whether a number of risk factors (such as smoking, overweight, etc.) are present or not.

Due to their huge costs it is unlikely that very large long-term cohort studies as in cardiovascular epidemiology will be performed in CAM research. However, moderately large prospective studies without a control group or non-randomized comparisons are, in principle, also cohort studies, and can to some extent be used for etiological or prognostic investigations. Here is an overlap between the classical epidemiological approach and the typical clinical research world.

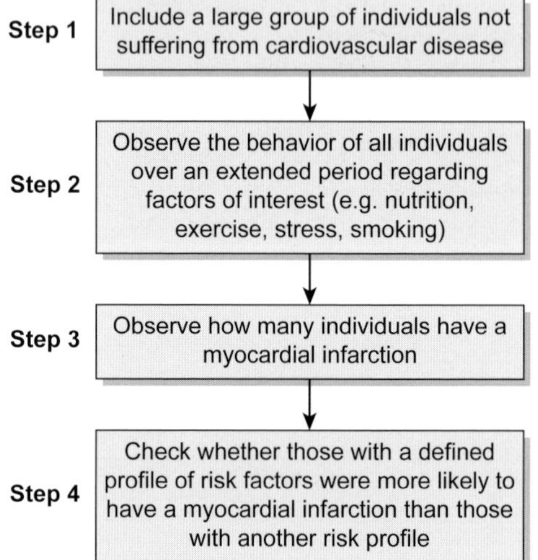

Fig. 11.5 Principle of a cohort study – A group of individuals not suffering from cardiovacsular disease is followed over an extended period of time to investigate the influence of risk factors on the likelihood of having a myocardial infarction

Cohort study – Example 7

Fung TT, Malik V, Rexrode KM, Manson JE, Willett WC, Hu FB. Sweetened beverage consumption and risk of coronary heart disease in women. Am J Clin Nutr. 2009;89:1,037–42.
Background: Previous studies have linked full-calorie sugar-sweetened beverages (SSBs) with greater weight gain and an increased risk of type 2 diabetes. Within a major cohort study the association between consumption of SSBs and the risk of coronary heart disease (CHD) in women was examined.

Methods: Women (n = 88,520) from the Nurses' Health Study aged 34–59 y, without previously diagnosed coronary heart disease (CHD), stroke, or diabetes in 1980, were followed from 1980 to 2004. Consumption of SSBs was derived from 7 repeated food-frequency questionnaires administered between 1980 and 2002. Relative risks (RRs) for CHD were calculated by using Cox proportional hazards models and adjusted for known cardiovascular disease risk factors.
Results: During 24 years of follow-up, 3,105 incident cases of CHD (nonfatal myocardial infarction and fatal CHD) were ascertained. After standard and dietary risk factors were adjusted for, the RRs (and 95 % CIs) of CHD according to categories of cumulative average of SSB consumption (< 1/mo, 1–4/mo, 2–6/wk, 1/d, and > or = 2 servings/d) were 1.0, 0.96 (0.87, 1.06), 1.04 (0.95, 1.14), 1.23 (1.06, 1.43), and 1.35 (1.07, 1.69) (P for trend < 0.001). Additional adjustment for body mass index, energy intake, and incident diabetes attenuated the associations, but they remained significant. Artificially sweetened beverages were not associated with CHD.
Conclusion: Regular consumption of SSBs is associated with a higher risk of CHD in women, even after other unhealthful lifestyle or dietary factors are accounted for.

FURTHER READING

Fletcher RW, Fletcher SW. Clinical epidemiology. The essentials. 4th edition. Philadelphia: Lippincott, Williams & Wilkins, 2005.

Knottnerus JA, Buntinx F. The Evidence Base of Clinical Diagnosis: Theory and Methods of Diagnostic Research. John Wiley & Sons, 2008.

Rothman KJ, Greenland S, Lash TL. Modern Epidemiology. Philadelphia: Lippincott, Williams & Wilkins, 2005.

Rothman KJ. Epidemiology: An Introduction. Oxford: Oxford University Press, 2002.

Appendix

Case studies

Case study 1: Uncontrolled observational study (pilot study)

Description: Case study 1 was a descriptive, observational study without control group, evaluating a treatment with special acupuncture needles that are left in situ for 7 days, an uncommon procedure but one frequently used by one particular acupuncturist.

Motivation: Andrew, an experienced acupuncturist, recently developed a new type of acupuncture needle that can be left in place for several days on the patient's back. Using these needles he saw very good results in a number of patients suffering from chronic low back pain. Since he sees many chronic pain patients in his practice, he wanted to evaluate the new technique. He had some advice on the study from a methodologist at the local university but he had no major funding source for his research.

Study question: Does pain decrease in patients suffering from chronic low back pain when they receive the newly developed acupuncture treatment?

Setting: Single center study, i.e. one acupuncture practice

Intervention: Patients received one session with retained needles. The acupuncture points were chosen according to the Chinese medicine pattern diagnosis and the needles were left in place for 7 days.

Control group: None

Co-interventions: Not predefined, but any additional treatments were documented throughout the study.

Randomization: Uncontrolled study – no randomization

Blinding: Uncontrolled study – no blinding

Inclusion criteria: Aged 18 years and above; clinical diagnosis of chronic low back pain with duration > 3 months and on average at least 40 mm pain on a visual analoque scale, and written informed consent

Exclusion criteria: None defined

Outcome measures: Low Back Pain (LBP) intensity measured on a visual analogue scale (VAS; 0–100 mm), back function questionnaire (HFAQ), quality of life questionnaire (SF-36), safety (adverse effects), satisfaction with treatment

Measurement time points: Baseline, two, six, and 12 months

Sample size: 40

Analysis population: all patients who were included in the study and who provided at least baseline data.

Data analysis: The statistical analysis was primarily descriptive; the statistical significance of changes between baseline and follow up was determined on an exploratory level (repeated measurement ANOVA). The primary analysis included all available data and in a further sensitivity analysis missing data were replaced by the last value carried forward method.

Results: 40 patients (mean ± SD age 57.2 ± 7.8 years, 67 % female) with an average disease duration of 12.5 ± 10.7 years were included in the study. The pain intensity measured on the VAS decreased from 61.1 ± 12.1 to 36.5 ± 27.4 mm after two months and this effect was nearly maintained at 12 months. A similar improvement was found for other parameters such as back function and quality of life.

Interpretation and conclusion: Patients suffering from chronic low back pain who received a single acupuncture treatment with needles retained for seven days had less back pain, better back function and a higher quality of life after two, six and 12 months compared to baseline. To evaluate whether this effect is caused by the novel acupuncture technique itself, a randomized controlled study would be necessary.

Case study 2: Randomized double-blind placebo-controlled study

Description: Case study 2 was an efficacy study. The objective of this randomized controlled trial was to evaluate whether a herbal medicininal product containing an extract from Harpagophytum procumbens (Devil's claw) given for two months is more effective than placebo in patients with chronic low back pain.

Motivation: Betty is working in a university outpatient center specialized in treating pain patients. She and two other colleagues are trained in herbal medicine. They noticed that patients suffering from chronic low back pain seemed to benefit from Devil's claw and reported their observation at several regional pain meetings. This triggered a discussion whether herbal medicine should become more systematically integrated into other units as well. However, a number of academics criticized this idea because there was not enough evidence that Devil's claw was effective when compared to placebo. They argued that it needed to be tested in a double-blind placebo-controlled trial. Betty was really keen to prove this and her boss supported her and suggested using the study as her PhD thesis.

Study question: Do patients who suffer from chronic low back pain experience better pain relief with Devil's claw than with placebo?

Setting: Multi-center trial with five university outpatient pain clinics

Intervention: 1,500 mg (1 coated tablet of 750 mg twice per day) of dried alcoholic extract of Harpagophytum procumbens over 2 months.

Control: Placebo (1 coated tablet twice per day, identical in appearance, taste and smell as the verum intervention)

Co-interventions: Patients were allowed to treat chronic low back pain with oral non-steroidal anti-inflammatory drugs, if required. The use of corticosteroids or pain-relieving drugs that act through the central nervous system was prohibited. All co-interventions were documented.

Randomization: Computer generated block randomization (ratio 1:1), identically packed sequentially numbered drug containers

Blinding: Patients, physicians and statistician blinded

Sample size: 140 patients (70 Devil's claw and 70 placebo)

Inclusion criteria: Aged 40 to 75 years; clinical diagnosis of chronic low back pain, duration > 6 months; average pain intensity of 40 or more on a 100-mm VAS during the last seven days; use of oral non-steroidal anti-inflammatory drugs only for pain treatment in the four weeks prior to treatment.

Exclusion criteria: Protrusion or prolapse of 1 or more intervertebral discs with concurrent neurological symptoms; radicular pain; prior vertebral column surgery; infectious spondylopathy; low back pain caused by inflammatory, malignant, or autoimmune disease; congenital deformation of the spine (except for slight lordosis or scoliosis); compression fracture caused by osteoporosis; spinal stenosis; spondylolysis or spondylolisthesis.

Outcome measures: Primary outcome measure: average LBP intensity of the last 7 days measured on a VAS (0–100 mm), secondary outcome measures: back function (HFAQ), quality of life (SF-36), days with pain medication (diary with drug and dosage); safety (AE and SAE).

Measurement time points: Baseline, two months, six months.

Analysis population: All patients who were randomized and provided baseline values

Data analysis: For the primary outcome (the reduction of the average pain intensity between baseline and two months on the 100 mm VAS) an ANCOVA adjusted for baseline values was used. Missing data were multiply imputed using regression methods.

Results: A total of 140 patients (67.8 % female; age 59 ± 9 years) were randomized (69 to Devil's claw group and 71 to placebo group). The average reduction in pain intensity after 2 months was 28.7 ± 30.3 mm (mean ± SD) in the devils claw group compared to 23.6 ± 31.0 mm in the placebo group (baseline adjusted difference between groups 5.1 mm and 95 % CI -3.7 to 13.9, p = 0.057).

Interpretation and conclusion: We found a non-significant reduction in patients with chronic low back pain who received devils claw compared to patients who received placebo.

Case study 3: Pragmatic randomized study comparing three groups

Description: Case study 3 was a comparative effectiveness study in a usual care setting. The objective of this pragmatic, randomized three-armed trial was to evaluate whether acupuncture treatment or yoga given in addition to usual care was more effective than usual care alone in the management of patients with chronic low back pain and whether one of these two treatments was more effective than the other.

Motivation: After completing medical school and training as an acupuncturist Carol earned a PhD in clinical epidemiology and was afterwards working at a CAM research department. She did observational studies of acupuncture for premenstrual syndrome and for low back pain, and ran a randomized trial of acupuncture for neck pain. The Ministry for Research had launched a program open for funding applications of comparative effectiveness research in patients with low back pain and Carol received a grant.

Study question: Do patients suffering from chronic low back pain who receive acupuncture or yoga in addition to usual care experience better pain relief than patients who receive usual care alone?

Setting: Multi-center trial in 30 GP practices, 20 acupuncture practices and 10 yoga centres

Intervention 1: Individualized acupuncture of up to 12 sessions given within 3 months, in addition to usual care.

Intervention 2: 12 Viniyoga sessions (90 min per session, one session per week, following the curriculum of the individual center) within 3 months, in addition to usual care

Control group: Usual care only.

Co-interventions: Both intervention groups were allowed to receive usual care. Patients in the control group received neither acupuncture nor yoga.

Randomization: computer generated central randomization (1:1:1), stratified for center, permuted block size.

Blinding: Open study – no blinding

Inclusion criteria: Aged 18 years and above; clinical diagnosis of chronic low back pain with a disease duration of > 6 months.

Exclusion criteria: Protrusion or prolapse of one or more intervertebral discs with concurrent neurologic symptoms; prior vertebral column surgery; infectious spondylopathy; low back pain caused by inflammatory, malignant, or autoimmune disease; compression fracture caused by osteoporosis.

Outcome measures: Primary outcome measure: back function (HFAQ) secondary outcome measures: quality of life (SF-36), days with pain medication (diary with drug and dosage), safety (AE and SAE).

Measurement time points: Baseline, 3 months, 6 months, 12 months

Sample size: 600 patients (200 acupuncture, 200 yoga, 200 usual care)

Analysis population: All randomized patients who provided baseline values

Data analysis: To determine differences between the intervention groups and the control group after 3 months ANCOVA adjusted for baseline values and center was used. Because of two primary analyses (acupuncture vs. usual care and yoga vs. usual care) Bonferroni correction was used to address the problem of multiple testing (i.e. an alpha of 0.025 was used as a significance level for each test). The difference between acupuncture and yoga was tested on a confirmatory basis because both interventions differed statistically significantly from usual care (hierarchical test procedure).

Results: A total of 600 patients (mean age 52.9 ± 13.7 years, 57.3 % female) were randomized (200 acupuncture, 200 yoga group and 200 usual care only).

Back function (HFAQ) at three months was 74.1 (95 % CI 73.0–75.2) in the acupuncture group, 74.6 (74.2–75.1) in the yoga group and 65.5 (64.3–66.7) in the usual care only group. A significant difference was found between acupuncture vs. usual care and yoga vs. usual care groups, $p< 0.001$, however no significant difference was found between yoga and acupuncture, $p = 0.806$).

Interpretation and conclusion: Patients with chronic low back pain, who received additional acupuncture or yoga treatment, experienced statistically significantly better back function after three months compared to patients who received only usual care. No significant difference was observed between the acupuncture and the yoga group.

Exercises: Formulating PICO questions

In the following original abstracts identify first the Patients (P), Intervention (I), Control (C) and Outcome (O). Try then to formulate a full research question including these four elements.

We have proposed solutions but, obviously, slightly different phrasing can be adequate as well, particularly if studies tend to be more pragmatic.

Example 1: Herbal medicine – efficacy of hawthorn (Crataegus) extract

Background: Crataegus preparations have been used for centuries especially in Europe. To date, no proper data on their efficacy and safety as an add-on-treatment are available. Therefore a large morbidity/mortality trial was performed.

Aim: To investigate the efficacy and safety of an add-on treatment with Crataegus extract WS 1,442 in patients with congestive heart failure.

Methods: In this randomised, double-blind, placebo-controlled multicenter study, adults with NYHA class II or III CHF and reduced left ventricular ejection fraction (LVEF< or = 35 %) were included and received 900 mg/day WS 1,442 or placebo for 24 months. Primary endpoint was time until first cardiac event.

Results: 2,681 patients (WS 1,442 : 1,338; placebo: 1,343) were randomised. Average time to first cardiac event was 620 days for WS 1,442 and 606 days for placebo (event rates: 27.9 % and 28.9 %, hazard ratio (HR): 0.95, 95 % CI [0.82; 1.10]; p = 0.476). The trend for cardiac mortality reduction with WS 1,442 (9.7 % at month 24; HR: 0.89 [0.73; 1.09]) was not statistically significant (p = 0.269). In the subgroup with LVEF> or = 25 %, WS 1,442 reduced sudden cardiac death by 39.7 % (HR 0.59 [0.37; 0.94] at month 24; p = 0.025). Adverse events were comparable in both groups.

Conclusions: In this study, WS 1,442 had no significant effect on the primary endpoint. WS 1,442 was safe to use in patients receiving optimal medication for heart failure. In addition, the data may indicate that WS 1,442 can potentially reduce the incidence of sudden cardiac death, at least in patients with less compromised left ventricular function.

Proposed solution

P	Patients with congestive heart failure (NYHA class II or III)
I	Hawthorn (Crataegus extract WS 1,442)
C	Placebo
O	Time until first cardiac event

Research question: Does the time until the first cardiac event differ between patients with congestive heart failure (NYHA class II or III) receiving either hawthorn (Crataegus extract WS 1,442) or a placebo?

REFERENCES

Holubarsch CJ, Colucci WS, Meinertz T, Gaus W, Tendera M; Survival and Prognosis: Investigation of Crataegus Extract WS 1,442 in CHF (SPICE) trial study group. The efficacy and safety of Crataegus extract WS 1,442 in patients with heart failure: the SPICE trial. Eur J Heart Fail. 2008 Dec; 10(12):1,255–63. Epub 2008 Nov 18.

Example 2: Efficacy of electro-acupuncture for preventing post-operative ileus

Aim: To examine whether acupuncture can prevent prolonged postoperative ileus (PPOI) after intraperitoneal surgery for colon cancer.

Methods: Ninety patients were recruited from the Fudan University Cancer Hospital, Shanghai, China. After surgery, patients were randomized to receive acupuncture (once daily, starting on postoperative day 1, for up to six consecutive days) or usual care. PPOI was defined as an inability to pass flatus or have a bowel movement by 96 h after surgery. The main outcomes were time to first flatus, time to first bowel movement, and electrogastroenterography. Secondary outcomes were quality of life (QOL) measures, including pain, nausea, insomnia, abdominal distension/fullness, and sense of well-being.

Results: No significant differences in PPOI on day 4 (P = 0.71) or QOL measures were found between the groups. There were also no group differences when the data were analyzed by examining those whose PPOI had resolved by day 5 (P = 0.69) or day 6 (P = 0.88). No adverse events related to acupuncture were reported.

Conclusion: Acupuncture did not prevent PPOI and was not useful for treating PPOI once it had developed in this population.

Proposed solution

P	Patients undergoing intraperitoneal surgery for colon cancer
I	Electro-acupuncture (once daily, starting on postoperative day 1, for up to six
	consecutive days)
C	Usual care
O	Prolonged postoperative ileus (inability to pass flatus or have a bowel movement by
	96 h after surgery)

Research question: Can acupuncture prevent prolonged postoperative ileus (PPOI) after intraperitoneal surgery for colon cancer more effectively than usual care (alone*)?

*Judging from the abstract it is unclear whether electro-acupuncture was given in addition to usual care or as an alternative (we assume the first).

REFERENCES

Meng ZQ, Garcia MK, Chiang JS, Peng HT, Shi YQ, Fu J, Liu LM, Liao ZX, Zhang Y, Bei WY, Thornton B, Palmer JL, McQuade J, Cohen L. Electro-acupuncture to prevent prolonged postoperative ileus: a randomized clinical trial. World J Gastroenterol. 2010 Jan 7; 16(1):104–11.

Example 3: Effectiveness of classical homeopathy and conventional therapy for atopic dermatitis

Background: One of five children visiting a homoeopathic physician is suffering from atopic eczema.

Objective: To examine the effectiveness, safety and costs of homoeopathic versus conventional treatment in usual care.

Methods: In a prospective multicentre comparative observational non-randomised study, 135 children (homoeopathy n = 48 vs. conventional n = 87) with mild to moderate atopic eczema were included. The primary outcome was the SCORAD (Scoring Atopic Dermatitis) at 6 months. Further outcomes at 6 and 12 months also included quality of life of parents and children, use of conventional medicine, treatment safety and disease-related costs.

Results: The adjusted SCORAD showed no significant differences between the groups at both 6 months (homoeopathy 22.49 + or − 3.02 [mean + or − SE] vs. conventional 18.20 + or − 2.31, p = 0.290) and 12 months (17.41 + or − 3.01 vs. 17.29 + or − 2.31, p = 0.974). Adjusted costs were higher in the homoeopathic than in the conventional group: for the first 6 months EUR 935.02 vs. EUR 514.44, p = 0.026, and for 12 months EUR 1,524.23 vs. EUR 721.21, p = 0.001. Quality of life was not significantly different between both groups.

Conclusion: Taking patient preferences into account, homoeopathic treatment was not superior to conventional treatment for children with mild to moderate atopic eczema.

Possible solution

P	Children with mild to moderate atopic eczema
I	Classical homeopathy
C	Usual care
O	SCORAD (Scoring Atopic Dermatitis) at 6 momths

Research question: Do children suffering from mild to moderate atopic eczema receiving classical homoeopathy have lower* symptom severity (SCORAD = Scoring Atopic Dermatitis) at six months than children receiving conventional treatment.

REFERENCES

Witt CM, Brinkhaus B, Pach D, Reinhold T, Wruck K, Roll S, Jäckel T, Staab D, Wegscheider K, Willich SN. Homoeopathic versus conventional therapy for atopic eczema in children: medical and economic results. Dermatology. 2009;219(4):329–40. ePub 2009 Oct 13.

Index

Notes

Notes

Notes

Notes